Eliciting Sounds
Techniques and Strategies for Clinicians

2nd Edition

Wayne A. Secord
The Ohio State University

Suzanne E. Boyce
University of Cincinnati

JoAnn S. Donohue
The Ohio State University

Robert A. Fox
The Ohio State University

Richard E. Shine
East Carolina University

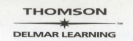

Eliciting Sounds: Techniques and Strategies for Clinicians, Second Edition

by Wayne A. Secord, Suzanne E. Boyce, JoAnn S. Donohue, Robert A. Fox, and Richard E. Shine

Vice President, Health Care Business Unit:
William Brottmiller

Director of Learning Solutions:
Matthew Kane

Senior Acquisitions Editor:
Sherry Dickinson

Product Manager:
Juliet Steiner

Editorial Assistant:
Angela Doolin

Marketing Director:
Jennifer McAvey

Marketing Manager:
Chris Manion

Marketing Coordinator:
Vanessa Carlson

Production Director:
Carolyn Miller

Content Project Manager:
Stacey Lamodi

Art Director:
Jack Pendleton

Library of Congress Cataloging-in-Publication Data

Eliciting sounds : techniques and strategies for clinicians / Wayne A. Secord ... [et al.]. -- 2nd ed.
    p. ; cm.
  Rev. ed. of: Eliciting sounds / Wayne Secord. c1981.
  Includes bibliographical references.
  ISBN-13: 978-1-4018-9725-3 (softbound : alk. paper)
  ISBN-10: 1-4018-9725-8 (softbound : alk. paper) 1. Speech therapy--Exercises--Handbooks, manuals, etc. I. Secord, Wayne. II. Secord, Wayne. Eliciting sounds.
  [DNLM: 1. Speech Therapy--methods--Handbooks. 2. Articulation Disorders--therapy--Handbooks. 3. Phonetics--Handbooks. WL 39 E42 2007]
  RC423.S38 2007
  616.85'506--dc22

                          2006103501

Notice to the Reader

Contents

Preface

At one time or another, most speech-language clinicians have experienced the frustration when they have attempted to elicit new speech sound behaviors. We not only feel this frustration in ourselves: we observe it in our clients as well. This is especially true when a young child or client does not have a target sound in his or her response repertoire, either imitatively or in contextual testing. We literally grasp for straws—searching for that one trick or technique that works. It was exactly one of these situations that led to the development of this book more than 25 years ago.

Like its predecessor, *Eliciting Sounds: Techniques and Strategies for Clinicians, Second Edition*, is designed to provide the clinician with a quick, easy-to-use array of techniques for quickly evoking any phoneme targeted for remediation. It also includes a description of place, manner, and voicing features, and a list of common errors for each of 42 phonemes. Every attempt has been made to keep the explanations of techniques short and simple and to provide as many techniques as possible for eliciting the more frequently misarticulated phonemes. We hope this book will be a valuable asset in therapy as well as a remedy for some of those frustrating sessions we've all experienced.

Acknowledgements

A number of professionals assisted in the development of the second edition of this work. I owe a great deal of gratitude to all of them for their hard work, commitment, and continued support. We had a real vision for the second edition, one that involved getting the science right, but just as importantly, making the book something extremely practical that any clinician could use. Good practice to me has always been just that: a mixture of good science and solid clinical skills. To that end, let me thank a few people who made all of this happen.

First, let me thank Suzanne Boyce and Rich Shine for giving us some new insights into our most problematic articulation errors. In this revision, we wanted clinicians to have a more in-depth understanding of the ever elusive /r/ and /ɚ/ and more specific guidelines for working with different types of lisping behaviors. Suzanne is a leading speech scientist who knows more about /r/ and /ɚ/ than anyone I know. I recall the day in Suzanne's speech science lab when she showed me more than 20 ultrasound images of acoustically correct productions of /ɚ/. Then she quickly pointed out that each of images represented a different tongue position. I saw the clinical relevance of her research immediately—that there was no single right way to make an /r/ sound. Rich and I have worked together for many years. We have similar backgrounds in motor speech that have been heavily influenced by Dr. Eugene McDonald at Penn State. Few clinicians understand the motor characteristics associated with lisping better than Rich. Thanks to both of you (Suzanne and Rich) for giving us some new knowledge and skills, but more importantly, for providing the clinical leverage to make a difference with so many children.

I would also like to thank my colleagues from The Ohio State University, Rob Fox and Jo Ann Donohue. They both worked tirelessly to check the material in this book. Rob handled his co-author responsibilities with precision and clarity. Rob is the poster child for "theory into practice." He was also our "Science Editor," ensuring that all scientific information was accurate as it could be, while enjoying the practical part of making those facts clinically relevant. In a book like this one really needs people who can think that way. Jo Ann and I go back a long way—to phonetics class at Ohio State. We were even "student teachers" in the schools at the same time. Except for the fact that she went to work with Dr. Van Riper, we were essentially raised in the same clinical world. We look at the clinical process similarly, and frankly, I cannot imagine revising this book without Jo Ann as a co-author. The clinical "good sense" properties of this book are directly attributable to Jo Ann. Thanks Rob and Jo Ann.

The first edition of *Eliciting Sounds* was published by Charles E. Merrill in 1981, a wonderful publisher. I will be forever indebted to Tom Hutchinson and Sandy Smith for encouraging a young author and seeing the value of a few good techniques for speech-language clinicians. Francie Margolin also played an important editorial and "co-author" role in the developmental process of the first edition. Like all great editors, Francie had the gift of clarity, something that often takes academic authors, I assure you, years to acquire.

For this edition, I continue to have support of a dynamic and creative publisher. I want to thank Kalen Conerly of Thomson Delmar Learning for believing in this project from the beginning. Like any great coach, she is always encouraging and has the patience of a saint. Juliet Steiner, our Product Manager, helped bring the book together. It is impossible to imagine what it is like to work with phonetic fonts, drawings, and other graphics. Juliet's competent management of the entire project, her clear thinking, and her sense of humor made the work so much easier. We also want to thank Matt McAdams for his illustrations and his unending patience with authors who insist that every illustration of the tongue had to be in exactly the right place. I want to thank everyone at Thomson Delmar Learning who worked so hard to ensure our success.

Many of the techniques contained in *Eliciting Sounds, Second Edition*, have been in use for years; but many are new. It would be impossible to trace their origin as they appear in one form or another in several articles and texts. As a result, we have chosen to cite only a few individuals whose techniques, strategies, or clinical concepts are recent enough that they can claim authorship of them. We would like to acknowledge several phonological researchers and master clinicians who have shared their work in professional publications, provided suggestions directly to us, or otherwise helped to shape the clinical concepts in this book. Thanks to all of you:

Merle Ansberry	Candace L. Goldsworthy	Roger McCabe
Nicholas W. Bankson	Mary Gordon	Eugene McDonalld
Anthony Bashir	Pamela Grunwell	Leija McReynolds
Judith Bauman-Wangler	Sara Stinchfield Hawk	Robert Milisen
Nanci Bell	Sibley Haycock	Donald Mowrer
Barbara H. Bernhardt	M. N. Hedge	Elizabeth McGinly Nemoy
John E. Bernthal	Barbara W. Hodson	Janet A. Norris
Mildred F. Berry	Paul Hoffman	Mardel Ogilvie
Ken M. Bleile	David Ingram	Leslie Olswang
Char Boshart	Ruth Beckey Irwin	Elaine Paden
Doris Bradley	Clint Johnson	Jayne Hall Parker
Anna Carr	Laura Justice	Adriana Pena-Brooks
Hugh Catts	Alan G. Kamhi	Karen Pollock
Nancy Creaghead	Lou Kennedy	Tom Powell
Serena Foley Davis	Ray Kent	Jo-Anne Prendeville
William Diedrich	Linda Khan	Froma Roth
Alice Dyson	Edward S. Klein	Ralph Shelton
Mary Louise Edwards	Joan Kwiatkowski	Larry Shriberg
Jon Eisenson	John Locke	Ann Bosma Smit
Mary Elbert	Robert Lowe	Ronald Sommers
Marc Fey	Harold Lillywhite	Carney Sotto
Hilda B. Fisher	Patricia Lindamood	Carol Stoel-Gammon
Ann Flowers	Phyllis Lindamood	Edith Strand
Judith Gierut	Daniel Ling	Linda Swank
Gail Gillon	Pam Marshalla	Mildred Templin
Ronald Goldman	Julie Masterson	James Torgeson

Ann Tyler	Curtis Weiss	Harris Winitz
Shelly Velleman	Robert West	Colleen K. Worthington
Fred Weiner	A. Lynn Williams	Edna Hill Young

Before the *Dedication* that follows, I would like to make two very personal acknowledgements. To my best friends since elementary school, Wally (Bubby) Jaynes and Tim Smith, thanks for more than 50 years of thoughtful "evidenced-based advice." We lost Bubby to pancreatic cancer a few years ago, but like children, Tim and I press on in our never-ending quest to change the world. Lastly, and most importantly, let me thank my wife Suzanne ("Suzy") for her love, sense of humor, and endless faith in me. We are quite a team, one hand, one heart.

Dedication

I would like to dedicate *Eliciting Sounds, Second Edition*, to Dr. Charles Van Riper of Western Michigan University. Dr. Van Riper's work inspired me greatly as a student. As a beginning clinician, I founded my practice on his principles of functionality. Since then, I have continued to stress that clinical practice boils down to empowering clients to use the skills they already have. Indeed, I have spent a lifetime teaching these principles to my own students and speech-language clinicians, i.e., *with and through others*. This book is testimony to Dr. Van Riper's influence, because it was truly developed with and through others.

Several years ago, when I was a junior faculty member at Ohio State, I received a letter from Dr. Van Riper. It scared me to death. Just imagine taking a letter out of *your* mailbox with the handwritten name of the one professor you idolize the most in the upper left-hand corner—*C. Van Riper*! To set the context a little more, consider the fact that less than a month before, I had presented a workshop on collaborative-consultation in the western part of Michigan, where I had told a large audience that I was indeed "Completely Van Riperized." Needless to say, despite the fact that my little joke was said with the utmost respect (of course), I was a bit concerned about why one of the founding fathers of our field might be writing to me—me! It took me several hours that day to get the nerve to actually open the letter. I would like to share that letter with you (see the following page for the letter). Today, I often read it to workshop participants, and for sure, not a single graduate student ever leaves the university without hearing "Dr. Secord's letter from Van Riper." Enjoy!

So now you know a little more about how and why the traditional approach to articulation therapy got started. But better than that, you get a chance to read the words of a clinical leader who took the time to pat someone else on the back. You hear his humility and feel his leadership and impact on our discipline. I tell my students some very similar things. Do what's best for your client! Take risks! Stick your neck out! And, most importantly, don't be afraid to develop better methods of your own. The ideas in this book are indeed only a map; the journey, as Van Riper said, is all yours.

Just one more thing: if you would ever want to see "Dr. Secord's letter from Van Riper," just stop in my office, and I'll show you its place on my wall—right next to my buckeye flag.

Wayne Secord

Department of Speech Pathology and Audiology
Charles VanRiper Language, Speech and Hearing Clinic

Kalamazoo, Michigan 49008-3825
616 387-8045

WESTERN MICHIGAN UNIVERSITY

September 26, 1993

Dear Dr. Secord,

Authors of textbooks in speech pathology rarely get fan letters but this is one.

In the miserable process of preparing the revision of my old text *Speech Correction* for its 9th Edition (God help me), I have had to do a lot of reading at the age of 88 and most of it is poorly written. Not so with your chapter on the Traditional Approach to Articulation in the book you co-authored with Nancy Creaghead and Parley Newman. You are lucid, interesting, and I bet your students love you.

I thank you for your presentation of my approach to articulation therapy. I couldn't have done it better myself and will use it as a model in the new revision.

Perhaps, the only suggestion I have, and it's a trivial one, is that in your historical account of early approaches, you didn't mention the Travis—Rasmus stimulus therapy. Indeed, it was that which impelled me to design a better way because it bored me silly. All the clinician would do would be to ask the client to repeat after her, "See, saw, so, sue, Now say saw; See, say, saw, sue; now say sue." That would go on for an hour. They felt that such a bombardment would lead to error elimination, can you imagine that? Again, at the University of Minnesota, they had a box resembling an outhouse in which the client sat in darkness while the clinician strongly prolonged an /s/ sound through a funnel in the doorway. Gad, it was a wonder both clinician and client could retain their sanity. Yet a few clients did manage to eliminate their lisps that way, but as you could imagine, most of them did not.

Now here's another thing. Edna Hill-Young, not Sarah Stinchfield-Hawk, was the inventor of the motokinesthetic approach though they co-authored their work. Edna was a very skilled therapist who had soft loving hands as I discovered once when I challenged her to teach me how to trill an /r/ sound. She tried hard but failed. She had success in helping the client to identify features of a target sound and how it contrasts with the error, but her success was probably due to the stimulation she provided as she manipulated the jaw and lips and pushed on the abdomen to initiate airflow. She was a beautiful woman and having her hovering over you like that was also quite stimulating.

And oh, those interminable breathing exercises and tongue exercises, and drill, drill, drill. Although my chief interest was in stuttering, I just couldn't bear watching those early clinicians belaboring those children with such nonsense so I tackled the problem and came up with a more sensible and logical approach. Now it is called *traditional*, and as you say it still is widely practiced in one form or another. Personally, in actual therapy, I constantly violated all the precepts I promulgated in the text. Unto their needs was my motto and to heck with what Van Riper or anyone else says. Rarely did I make my clients climb that staircase step by step, and I constantly urged my students to develop better methods of their own. But one needs some kind of a map when you set out on a journey and I guess I provided one and not much more.

I would appreciate any suggestions regarding stuff that should be deleted or added when redoing my chapter. Well, sir, this has unexpectedly turned out to be a long letter, but at least you know you have a fan.

Yours,

Charles Van Riper

Chapter 1

Introduction

Eliciting Sounds: Techniques and Strategies for Clinicians, Second Edition, is a quick and comprehensive resource for speech language clinicians, providing a variety of strategies and techniques for teaching correct sound production of consonants, vowels, and diphthongs. *Eliciting Sounds, Second Edition,* focuses on the most frequently misarticulated sounds—the consonants—because of the wide variety of techniques for improving consonant sound production. Indeed, more than two-thirds of the book is devoted to the 24 English consonant phonemes. This text also emphasizes problematic articulation errors, including those that occur on the many variations of /r/, divided into two categories: pre-vocalic (consonant) /r/ and post-vocalic (vowel) /ɚ/. These types of errors occur often and are uniquely challenging for speech-language pathologists. In addition, the discussion of vowels and diphthongs focuses on typical errors and general strategies used to elicit correct production. Finally, *Eliciting Sounds, Second Edition,* concludes with three Appendices that present supplementary assessment and treatment information. Appendix A outlines detailed, step-by-step procedures for evaluating speech sound stimulability. Appendix B contains extensive word lists that can be used to evaluate articulation consistency and identify key words in which sounds are produced correctly. The "Quick

Screens" in Appendix B cover all English speech sounds except /ʒ/. Finally, in Appendix C, Dr. Richard Shine describes elicitation and early treatment procedures for addressing lisping behaviors. Building on other techniques for eliciting /s/ presented in the book, Appendix C is new to the second edition.

Background

The clinical management of articulation and phonology almost always begins with a complete assessment of the client's articulation response repertoire (sound system). The assessment indicates which sounds clients can say spontaneously, which ones they can produce imitatively, which ones they can produce in some but not all phonetic contexts, and which ones they cannot produce at all. After analyzing all assessment data, the clinician often recommends phonological intervention, and treatment typically focuses on training the client to say one or more of the error sounds correctly.

Treatment almost always begins by building upon what the client can already say or do (current perceptual and motor skills). The clinician examines each sound targeted for treatment and uses assessment data to decide where to begin. For example, if the client can already say a target sound some of the time (inconsistently) or can say it correctly in response to the clinician's auditory model (stimulation), the treatment process typically gets started quickly. The therapy essentially focuses on improving the client's overall accuracy or correctness and then moves to building fluency (production with ease and speed). Indeed, most therapies for articulation errors work this way. They begin with simple, less complex utterances (isolated sounds, syllables, or words) and move to more complex productions (contextually varied words, then phrases, sentences, and conversation). Phonological intervention requires careful clinical management, but most clinicians feel the process is much easier to manage when the client can already say or imitate the sound correctly. Step-by-step procedures for assessing a client's response to auditory and visual stimulation (speech sound stimulability) are provided in Appendix A.

Sometimes finding the right place to start therapy is more difficult. If the client cannot say the target sound correctly even some of the time and cannot imitate it, the clinician will need to find another place to start. The coarticulatory effects of adjacent sounds often make speech production easier in some words or contexts than others. So it is highly likely that the client will be able to say the target sound(s) correctly in some words or phonetic contexts. These "key words" (Van Riper, 1978) or "facilitating contexts" (McDonald, 1964) represent highly favorable phonetic environments in which the client can clearly produce the target sound correctly. One comprehensive program that clinicians can use to assess contextual variation is the *S-CAT: Secord Contextual Articulations Tests* (Secord and Shine, 2003). The *S-CAT* assessment materials allow the clinician to identify key words or contexts in which the client produces the target sound correctly and then use these stimuli in a variety of formats to increase accuracy and fluency on error sounds. Materials adapted from the *S-CAT* are included in Appendix B to help clinicians identify these key points of entry into the treatment process.

However, when the client cannot produce a target sound at all, such as in response to auditory stimulation (imitation) or in any key word or favorable phonetic context, the clinician must initially establish the correct production. In a matter of speaking, the clinician needs to "roll up her sleeves" and actually teach the client how to say the target sound. *Eliciting Sounds, Second Edition,* is designed with that purpose in mind. It is designed for use at the very beginning of articulation training (the establishment phase) for eliciting correct phoneme production in isolation, in syllables, or in words. *Eliciting Sounds, Second Edition,* provides many techniques for establishing correct production of individual sounds.

Methods for Eliciting Sounds

Let us now take a look at some popular methods for eliciting sounds. In this book, a *method* refers to a larger overall approach, and a *technique* refers to a specific procedure used to evoke production of one or more phonemes. In addition, discussion of children's error patterns uses the term *strategy* to mean a conceptual tactic or clinical orientation that can be used to approach error patterns. For each target sound, *Eliciting Sounds, Second Edition,* begins by describing techniques based on imitation and use of context; however, the book also focuses on methods and techniques that can be used when the client cannot produce a target sound at all.

Imitation

Several authors suggest that imitation should be the first method used to elicit new sounds (Bernthal and Bankson, 2004; Bauman-Waengler, 2004; Creaghead, Neuman, and Secord, 1989; Gordon-Brannan and Weiss, 2007; Van Riper, 1978; Van Riper and Emerick, 1984). Imitation, also known traditionally as *auditory stimulation*, requires the client to repeat a target sound after the clinician has presented one or more examples. Even when the client is not stimulable in the initial assessment, the clinician may be able to use imitation as a first step in training. Auditory stimulation is widely used and is probably the best-known technique for eliciting new sounds.

Imitation quite naturally combines with other methods for establishing new sounds. For example, a clinician might use a phonetic placement technique (described below) to help the client first produce the sound and then revert to imitation for practice. In subsequent sessions, the clinician might use both phonetic placement instruction and auditory stimulation.

Use of Context

Although assessment of articulation consistency is not actually a method for eliciting sounds, it is useful for identifying phonetic contexts in which a client can correctly produce a target sound. As with imitation, facilitating contexts can be used either as a beginning point for therapy or in combination with other techniques to develop accuracy and fluency. For example, if a client can produce a sound in a few contexts but cannot imitate it in other contexts, the clinician may begin with phonetic placement, then point out words where the client produces the sound correctly, and then provide practice on the available facilitating contexts. The clinician might also present models for imitation frequently throughout the session.

Phonetic Placement

Phonetic placement is one of the oldest approaches to eliciting sounds (Scripture and Jackson, 1927). The clinician instructs the client in the correct placement of the articulators, modification of the airstream (breath), and voicing. The goal of phonetic placement is to give the client as many clues as possible to the positioning of the articulators and the handling of the outgoing airstream. For example, clinicians use illustrations or diagrams of tongue or lip placement or movement, as well as applicators or instruments (e.g., tongue depressors, cotton swabs, etc.) to explain correct sound production. Gordon-Brannan and Weiss (2007, p. 195) summarize techniques and devices used in the phonetic placement method:

1. Tongue depressors to manipulate or hold the articulators in place

2. Manipulation of the articulators with the clinician's gloved fingers

3. Verbal descriptions or instructions

4. Airstream (breath) indicators for the mouth and nose

5. Graphic indicators (e.g., spectrograms)

6. Feeling the air stream with the hand or observing its effects on a tissue

7. Observing the clinician or self in a mirror while producing sounds

8. Feeling laryngeal vibration

9. Observing diagrams, pictures, or drawings of the articulators while producing sounds

10. Observing computer-based renderings of articulators while producing certain sounds.

However, these are only a few of the techniques that can be used alone or in combination in the phonetic placement method. The variety of available techniques is as great as the clinician's ability to invent new ones.

The Moto-Kinesthetic Method

The moto-kinesthetic method developed by Edna Hill-Young in the late 1930s is very similar to phonetic placement. While wearing latex gloves, the clinician places her own hands on the client's articulatory mechanism (usually the lips, jaw, or face) to direct the movements necessary for each speech sound. By manipulating these external articulators, the clinician draws the client's attention to the place at which movement begins, the amount of tension or pressure needed, the overall shape and direction of movement, and the timing. The clinician uses the tactile and kinesthetic senses to help the client feel the way the sound is produced. As the clinician directs the movements, she also provides visual and auditory stimulation to give the client a greater sensory impression of correct production. Most of the specific moto-kinestetic techniques presented in this book are derived from the work of Young and Hawk (1938, 1955). Although these stimulation techniques are now more than 50 years old, they are still clinically relevant and appropriate.

Sound Approximation

Sound approximation refers to two similar approaches—progressive approximation and modification of other sounds—both of which involve the learning principle of *shaping* (Van Riper, 1978). In progressive approximation, the clinician stimulates the client to produce a series of sounds or sound segments that gradually approximate the target response, until the actual target sound is produced. Van Riper describes progressive approximation as follows:

> The clinician joins the client and makes the same error the client makes. She then shows the client a series of transitional sounds, each of which comes a bit closer to the standard sound until finally the standard sound is produced. Each little modification the client makes that comes a bit closer to the goal is rewarded. Those variations that move away from the target sound are ignored. (1978, p. 188)

Thus, the clinician begins with the client's error and gradually modifies it, using her own finely tuned discrimination skills to guide the client's productions. Many clinicians are familiar with and use this method—for instance, with a client who has a distorted /ɚ/ which resembles the /ʊ/ in *put*. The client initially produces the error /ʊ/ in isolation and is guided by the clinician's instructions to produce sounds that come closer and closer to the target /ɚ/.

The second type of sound approximation method is modification of other sounds. Here the clinician uses another sound or sounds already in the client's repertoire as a point of departure for the target sound. The clinician instructs the client to produce a known sound and then to adjust the articulators in certain ways as he continues to produce the known sound. Each articulatory adjustment is a movement that comes closer to the position necessary for the target sound. This method is often used with non-speech sounds, such as coughing to elicit a /k/ or growling to elicit /ɚ/. Once the client produces a sound that is close to the target, the clinician can use other techniques, such as imitation and further phonetic placement instruction, to bring the client's production precisely on target.

Metaphors, Descriptions, Demonstrations, and Touch Cues

In his *Manual of Articulation and Phonological Disorders, Second Edition*, Bleile (2004) describes several categories of "facilitative techniques" that clinicians use to effect change in a client's articulation and phonological development. One of his major categories of facilitative techniques is called *metaphors, descriptions, demonstrations, and touch cues*. Clinicians can use metaphors (verbal comparisons, such as the "growling sound") to make the therapeutic process easier to understand, especially for young children. Descriptions and demonstrations provide a simpler, more straightforward way to heighten a child's awareness to the characteristics of speech that matter most. Touch cues work similarly: they focus the child's attention and provide a multi-sensory awareness of a target sound's phonetic properties (especially place of articulation). *Eliciting Sounds, Second Edition,* presents many of these facilitative techniques. One can also consider phonetic placement and sound approximation techniques as illustrative demonstrations that fit into Bleile's categories: they both use sensible descriptive language and often incorporate child-friendly language (metaphors) as well as touch cues to magnify the child or client's sensory image of a target sound's salient features.

Organization of *Eliciting Sounds, Second Edition*

Eliciting Sounds, Second Edition, is organized into the commonly accepted categories of speech sounds: consonants (Chapter 2), vowels (Chapter 3), and diphthongs (Chapter 4). There is also extensive coverage of prevocalic /r/ and postvocalic /ɚ/ (Chapter 5), as well as supplementary assessment and treatment information presented in the Appendices (A, B, and C).

Consonants

Chapter 2 covers techniques for eliciting consonant sounds. It begins with an overview of the place, manner, and voicing features used in producing consonant phonemes, followed by sections on specific consonants. The consonants are organized by manner of articulation in the following order: stops, fricatives, affricates, nasals, glides, and liquids. The discussion of each phoneme includes these elements:

1. A recap of the place/manner/voicing (PMV) features for that particular consonant.
2. A simple explanation of how the sound is produced.
3. A diagram illustrating the correct tongue or lip placement.
4. A list of common errors encountered by clinicians.
5. A list of contextual variations where appropriate.
6. A list of phonetic placement techniques to demonstrate the position of the articulators, the handling of the airstream, and the voicing characteristics.
7. A summary of the specific moto-kinesthetic stimulation prescribed for that phoneme.
8. A list of sound approximation techniques involving both progressive approximation and modification of other sounds.

Neither imitation nor use of context is discussed. However, supplementary information on imitation and use of context is provided in Appendix A and B, respectively. For more information on imitation or contextual utilization strategies, see current comprehensive articulation texts such as Bernthal and Bankson (2005) or Bauman-Wangler (2004). Information on strategies for contextual assessment is found in the original work of McDonald (1964) on the *S-CAT* developed by Secord and Shine (2003).

Vowels and Diphthongs

Chapters 3 and 4 provide an overview of the articulatory characteristics of vowels (monothongs and diphthongs). Chapter 3 discusses common vowel (monothong) errors and ways to produce each vowel, summarizes dialectal variations, and describes strategies for eliciting correct vowel production, including a summary of the moto-kinesthetic stimulations for each sound. Chapter 4 expands the discussion of vowels to cover diphthongs. The chapter opens by explaining the articulation of diphthongs—that is, how they result from the production of two vowels as a glide. The chapter then discusses common errors, dialectal variations, and general eliciting strategies.

Prevocalic and Postvocalic /ɚ/

Chapter 5 takes an in-depth look at /r/ and /ɚ/ (schwar) sound productions. Without a question, these sounds present the greatest challenge to speech-language clinicians. Indeed, some school-age children receive therapy for many years before their /r/ or /ɚ/ errors are corrected. Chapter 5 is designed to clear up a number of misconceptions about the production of /r/ or /ɚ/. It contains illustrations and examples of ways to produce /r/ and /ɚ/, along with an extensive list of techniques for successful starting points for this type of therapy.

Supplementary Information

The second edition of *Eliciting Sounds* provides new content that will assist clinicians in the assessment and treatment process. This information is arranged into three Appendices.

Appendix A: Speech Sound Stimulability

Appendix A provides step-by-step procedures for testing speech sound stimulability. Although this type of assessment is widely used, the authors feel the procedures vary considerably, and few resources described them in detail. The methodology presented in *Eliciting Sounds, Second Edition,* has been used with many children and may be very useful for students who are just beginning their clinical training experience.

Appendix B: Quick Screens of Articulation Consistency

Appendix B contains *Quick Screens (QS) of Articulation Consistency* for consonants, vowels, and diphthongs. Compiled from the *Secord Contextual Articulation Tests (S-CAT),* the *QS* materials provide clinicians with a quick estimate of phonetic variability (consistency) and an effective means to identify phonetic contexts in which the client articulates target sounds correctly. *QS* screening probes are provided for all consonants except /ʒ/, as well as all vowels and diphthongs.

Appendix C: Strategies for Treating Lisping Behaviors

In addition to the techniques and strategies provided for /s/ and /ʒ/, Appendix C provides additional information on the nature of lisping. Dr. Richard Shine identifies the three primary types of lisping behaviors and outlines a specific elicitation procedure that he has taught to student for years. Although the example described in detail is for the lateral /s/ lisp, the procedures work well for all three types of lisps. Illustrations are provided to augment the clear and precise explanation of the overall methodology.

A Word about Safety

Throughout *Eliciting Sounds, Second Edition,* many of the strategies and techniques suggest the use of tactile cues. Clinicians are encouraged to utilize universal precautions to promote adequate hygiene and prevent the transmission of communicable diseases. More often than not, this will generally require the use of latex gloves, dental swabs, tongue depressors, etc., and frequent washing of hands. Please be mindful of these precautions as you work with the client.

Conclusion

Welcome to *Eliciting Sounds, Second Edition.* This first chapter has explained the purpose of the book and presented some important overview information. It improves on the first edition and alternative textbooks in many ways. First, it is a mix of science and practice: it is phonetically precise, yet still very practical. Second, this edition has revised many older strategies and techniques presented in the first edition, as well as adding many new ones and organizing the information in a much more learner-friendly way. It has also made significant improvements in the artwork and other graphics used throughout the text. The new "art" is not only easy to understand but also extensive. Third, there is much more information on /s/ and /r, ɚ/ than ever before, with clearer discussion and more techniques. Finally, like the previous edition, *Eliciting Sounds, Second Edition,* presents all this information in a clear and useful way so that clinicians can provide the very best services for their clients.

Chapter 2

Consonant Sounds

Articulation of Consonants

Consonants are phonemes produced with a significant degree of constriction in the vocal tract. This constriction can range from a complete closure for stops to a partial occlusion for glides. The 24 consonants of English are traditionally classified according to three features: place of articulation, manner of articulation, and voicing. These major feature classifications and their characteristics are described in more detail below. However, *Eliciting Sounds, Second Edition*, consistently uses traditional terminology ("clinical descriptors"), such as *lips, teeth, tongue (tip, blade, front, back), front of the mouth, roof of the mouth,* and *back of the mouth,* for describing the common errors, and for suggesting techniques and strategies for eliciting correct sound productions.

Place of Articulation

Place of articulation refers to that point in the vocal tract where the articulators obstruct the outgoing airstream to produce the consonant sound. The term "articulators" refers to those portions of the vocal tract (such as the lips, teeth, and tongue) that produce the constrictions. The articulators may make complete contact, totally obstructing the airstream; they may approximate one another; or they may simply narrow the vocal tract. Figure 2.1 shows a cross section of the human vocal tract, indicating these specific places of articulation.

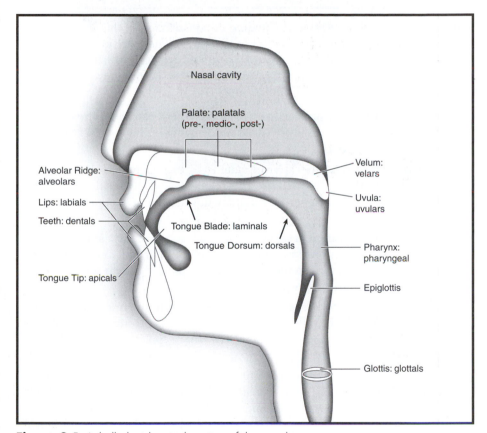

Figure 2.1 Labelled midsagittal section of the vocal tract

The place of articulation of any consonant sound refers to the point or points of the primary constriction of the vowel tract. For example, /s/ is a lingua-alveolar sound produced with the tongue raised to the alveolar ridge. However, this description does not provide any detail concerning which portion of the tongue is used as the articulator (tip or blade). A more specific description might be lingua (apical) alveolar (using the tongue tip) or lingua (laminal) alveolar (using the tongue blade). The /t/ in English is often produced with the apex of the tongue (tongue tip) directly contacting the alveolar ridge; thus, it would be considered an lingua (apical) alveolar sound. Similarly, /f/ is labiodental because contact is made between the lower lips and the upper teeth. Please note that many phonetics texts refer to the place of articulation of lingual sounds (e.g., lingua-dental, lingua-alveolar, lingua-palatal, lingua-velar) without the "lingua" term (e.g., dental, alveolar, palatal, velar).

Manner of Articulation

Manner of articulation refers to the degree of constriction of the vocal tract that occurs in the production of a consonant sound. There are six manners of articulation by which consonant sounds are classified, each of which is used to describe how groups of sounds are produced by obstructing the airstream in a similar way.

1. Stops: The articulators make contact to stop the airstream completely. The impounded air is then usually released suddenly with a burst of air (the "stop closure release"): /p, b, t, d, k, g/.

2. Fricatives: The articulators approximate to form a narrowed channel in the vocal tract through which the airstream passes. The result is a noisier sound that gives the listener an auditory impression of friction: /s, z, ʃ, ʒ, θ, ð, f, v, h/.

3. Affricates: An affricate represented the quick sequence of a stop and a fricative produced as one unit at the same place of articulation. The articulators make contact to stop the airstream completely, which they then release through a fricative opening: /tʃ, dʒ/.

4. Nasals: The articulators make a complete closure in the oral cavity while the velum is lowered to allow the airstream to pass through the nasal passages (through the nasopharyngeal port): /m, n, ŋ/.

5. Glides: The articulators move from one position to another. They are not as closely approximated as they are in the production of fricatives; but the vocal tract is more tightly constricted than it is for vowels. For this reason, these sounds are sometimes referred to as *approximates*. Glides have a considerable degree of resonance (as do vowels; hence, the term *semivowels*) because of the relatively wide opening of the vocal tract airstream: /w, j/.

6. Liquids: These sounds are very similar to glides in that they have considerable resonance and are not as closely approximated as fricatives. Liquids include two types of sounds: lateral sounds (/l/) and rhotic (r-colored) sounds (/r/). In lateral sounds, there is a complete closure in the central portion of the oral cavity (e.g., the tongue tip is pressed against the

alveolar ridge), but the airstream can flow through an opening on one or both sides of the tongue. Rhotic sounds—the /r/ sounds in English—also involve an approximation (but not an occlusion) between articulators but represent relatively complex articulations. For this reason, a complete chapter is devoted to rhotic sounds later in this text.

Voicing

Consonant sounds are either voiced or voiceless (unvoiced). A voiced consonant is produced with the vocal folds vibrating; a voiceless consonant, with no vibration.[1] Table 2.1 classifies the 24 consonants according to place of articulation, manner of articulation, and voicing. The voiced consonants are shaded. Cognates are pairs

Table 2.1 Features of Consonant Vowels						
Place			**Manner**			
	Stops	**Fricatives**	**Affricates**	**Nasals**	**Glides**	**Liquids**
Bilabial	p b			m	ʍ w*	
Labiodental		f v				
Apical-dental		θ ð				
Apical-alveolar	t d			n		l
Laminal-alveolar		s z				
Palato-alveolar		ʃ ʒ	tʃ dʒ			
Palatal					j	
Central-palatal						r
Velar	k g			ŋ	ʍ w	
Glottal	ʔ**	h				

The sounds /w/ and /ʍ/ are labio-velars.

***The glottal stop /ʔ/ does not constitute a separate phoneme in English and is not covered in Chapter 2.*

---

[1] Phonetically, the voiceless/voiced distinction in American English is often realized as an aspirated/unaspirated distinction, especially in syllable-initial positions. For example, in American English, an initial voiced stop (/b/, /d/, /g/) is often phonetically unvoiced during the stop closure itself (the occlusion phase) but has a very short voice onset time with no period of aspiration after the stop closure release. However, this book approaches voicing distinctions in stops from the point of view of producing maximal distinctions in the client; that is, we will seek to elicit initial voiced stops that are both voiced and unaspirated (these are sometimes called "prevoiced" stops), and voiceless stops that are both voiceless and unaspirated.

of consonants produced with the same place and manner of articulation that differ in regard to voicing. Cognate pairs appear in the same cell, with one possible exception. Some systems list /ʍ/ (also transcribed as /hw/) as a voiceless cognate of /w/. We have omitted /ʍ/ because it is only rarely used in current dialects of American speech (it is more common in Appalachian English that in other varieties of English). It will not be included in the discussion of eliciting techniques.

The following section examines individual consonant sounds. The consonants are organized by manner of articulation, beginning with stops and proceeding through to liquids. For each consonant, a section describes sound production, common articulation errors, and techniques for eliciting correct sounds. Use of a mirror is recommended for many of the techniques presented. Please note that the production descriptions assume that the sound is being produced in syllable-initial position. For each consonant, we will list a few of the phonetic variations (allophones) that are found in other phonetic contexts (including final position).

One Final Caution

The techniques described in this chapter often emphasize one articulatory gesture over another. As such, they may lead to confusion in the hearing impaired, causing these clients to overemphasize or adopt one particular gesture over another. The clinician is cautioned to consider the appropriateness of each technique when working with a hearing impaired individual.

/p/

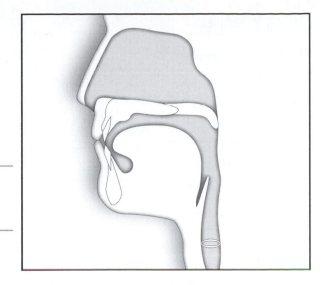

PMV Features:

Bilabial/stop/voiceless

Production:

The lips are brought together to obstruct the unvoiced airstream completely. The jaw is in a closed position to assist with the closure of the lips. The velum is raised so that intra-oral breath pressure can build up. The lips are then separated to allow the unvoiced air pressure to escape suddenly in the form of an aspirated (breathy) burst of energy.

Common Errors:

Voicing: b/p
Labiodental/fricative: f/p
Glottal/fricative: h/p
Glottal/stop: ?/p
Labiodental/stop (an unexploded /f/)
Excessive or insufficient plosion (explosion of air)
Omission

Common Contextual Variants:

Unrounded /p/: peep, pip, pat
Rounded /pʷ/: pool, pole, pull, Paul
Unaspirated /p⁼/: spin, spot
No audible release burst /p̚/: apt, uptown, cupcake

Eliciting Techniques:

Phonetic Placement

Demonstrate the feature characteristics of /p/:

- Bilabial placement (closure)
- Jaw position closed
- Breathy burst of air
- Velum closed
- Vocal folds silent

1. Instruct the client to close his mouth, fill up his cheeks with air and then blow out the air in short bursts. You may need to manually remind him to close his lips, puff out his cheeks.

2. Hold a small piece of string, a feather, or a small strip of lightweight paper about one inch from the client's mouth. Ask the client to make the string, feather, or paper move by (blowing), exploding the air out of the mouth. You may need to instruct the client to first close his mouth and fill up his cheeks with air, then tell him to blow.

3. Place a tongue depressor horizontally between the lips. Ask the client to close his lips on the tongue depressor and explode air.

4. Instruct the client to blow out in a sustained (long) breath. Then tell him to use his lips to break up the breath into shorter and shorter puffs (bursts) of air.

5. Demonstrate the explosive force of /p/ on the client's hand. The client then attempts to do the same thing with his hand.

6. Have the client attempt to spin a pinwheel with rapid productions of /p/. Draw attention to the bursts (force) of air. Press the lips together with your fingers, if necessary.

7. Use a cotton swab to lightly touch the surfaces of the lips where contact is made to explode the air. Instruct the client to bring the lips together to touch that spot, then blow puffs of air through the closed lips. Remind the clie nt that the air popped out of the mouth, rather than slipping or creeping out.

8. Tell the client to produce the motor-boat sound, the dripping sound, the popping sound, the kissing sound, or the "quiet brother" of /b/. (Lindamood and Lindamood, 1998).

Moto-Kinesthetic

Using latex gloves, the clinician places her thumb and forefinger on the client's lower jaw below the lower lip. The jaw is moved upward until it presses against the upper lip. The lower jaw is brought downward, quickly and firmly. The clinician should make sure that the lower jaw and lip motion is first directed upward to contact the upper lip and that this motion is then reversed to direct movement into the next speech sound.

   As a variation, she can also apply pressure to the lips with the thumb, forefinger, and index finger, then bring the lips together and apart in a slow-motion manner. The clinician demonstrates this technique first, then the client attempts it in front of the mirror. In either approach, the clinician should place her thumb on the client's cheek to discourage puffing of the cheeks and to encourage bilabial obstruction of the air stream.

Sound Approximation

1. Develop initial bilabial movements by comparing /p/ with silent /m/. Place a small hand mirror that has been chilled between the client's upper lip and the nose so that nasal emission during /m/ may be illustrated. The nostrils can also be lightly pinched to reduce accompanying nasality.

2. Instruct the client to produce /b/ /b/ /b/ and then turn off the vocal folds. For the younger child you may want to say "turn off the motor" or "don't make a buzzing sound—just blow air." Compare the amount of explosion needed for /p/ and /b/, since /p/ is more breathy (i.e., a more intense burst of energy) and is characterized by more tension.

3. Tell the client to prolong the /h/ sound while gradually closing the lips, and then continue the sound with the lips closed for a little longer to allow more air to fill the mouth. Finally, explode the air.

4. Instruct the client to kiss the back of his hand, and draw attention to the lip seal created. Tell the client to continue to make the kissing sound while moving the hand to his side and making the kiss sound more quietly. Repeat the kisses, emphasizing blowing air out instead of drawing air in.

/b/

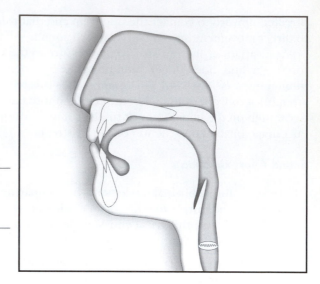

PMV Features:

Bilabial/stop/voiced

Production:

The voiced cognate of /p/, /b/ is produced simi- larly: The lips are pressed together to permit a com- plete stoppage of the airstream. Voicing begins and then the lips are parted to release the intra-oral breath pressure in the form of a sudden burst of energy, somewhat less aspirated (breathy), and less tense than /p/.

Common Errors:

1. Unvoicing: p/b
2. Labiodental/fricative: v/b
3. Glottal/fricative/unvoicing: h/b
4. Nasal: m/b
5. Insufficient pressure release
6. Omission

Common Contextual Variants:

Unrounded /b/: bean, bit, bait, but
Rounded /bʷ/: boot, bush, boat
No audible release burst /b˥/: cabs, curbside, rubdown

Eliciting Techniques:

Phonetic Placement

Demonstrate the feature characteristics of /b/:

- Lips coming together
- Jaw position closed
- Slight explosion of air
- Velum closed
- Voicing (Take the client's hand and place it on your throat while you say /b/.)

1. Place the flat surface of a tongue depressor between the lips so that both lips can hold it firmly. Have the client practice opening and closing the lips on the tongue depressor with equal pressure. Then tell the client to form a bilabial seal using the upper lip, the tongue depressor, and the lower lip. Tell the client to lightly force and hold air at the center of the lips or the center of the tongue depressor without puffing his cheeks. Tell the client to hold the tongue depressor more firmly, then quickly remove the tongue depressor. To coordinate voicing and plosive burst, hold one hand lightly on the client's throat as a reminder. Lightly touch the throat to institute voicing just before removing the tongue depressor.

2. Other demonstrations useful in describing the characteristics of /b/:

   a. Hold a small piece of lightweight paper or a feather in front of your mouth while you demonstrate the plosive release. It is most important that you demonstrate voicing before release. Tell a young child that "the motor comes on first."

   b. Place one of the client's hands on your throat while you demonstrate the plosive release of /b/ on his other hand. Then have the client do the same with you. When you demonstrate, press the client's hand lightly against your throat to show voicing before producing the /b/ on his hand.

   c. Remind the client to use the bubble sound, the dripping sound, the water-boiling sound, or the "noisy brother" of /p/ (Lindamood and Lindamood, 1998).

3. For additional eliciting techniques, please turn to the description of the consonant /p/. Make certain to adapt the directions so that you include the voiced component when eliciting /b/. Remind young children to "turn on the motor," "use your voice box," or "use the buzzing sound," or contrast the quiet and noisy sounds.

Moto-Kinesthetic

The moto-kinesthetic stimulation for /b/ differs slightly from that of /p/. For /b/, the clinician places the thumb and forefinger of one hand on the client's upper lip and the thumb and forefinger of the other hand on the client's lower lip. The clinician presses both lips together with equal force and then separates them. The clinician should note that in /p/ the upper lip is not touched; the lower lip is brought upward to contact the upper lip. In /b/, both lips are touched with equal pressure and then separated.

Sound Approximation

1. Shape /b/ from a prolonged /ʌ/ (or with /p/ if it is in the client's repertoire). Tell the client to prolong /ʌ/ and then stop the sound by closing both lips. T hen tell the client to do the same but much faster. What often results is /ʌbə, ʌbə, ʌbə/, from which /bə/ can be extracted (a voiced consonant is easier to elicit in the voiced intervocalic /V_V/ context)

2. Shape /b/ from /p/ by focusing attention to minimal contrasting aspect of voicing.

3. Shape /b/ from /m/ by instructing the client to explode an /m/. Here, however, the clinician is cautioned to demonstrate rather abrupt production of /mʌ, mʌ, mʌ/ and make them become /bə, bə, bə/ quickly so that she does not confuse the client. Often /m/ can be used easily with clients who understand plosive release as in /p/ but who cannot initiate voicing first as required for /b/. The client can be instructed to place his lips together for /m/, to say a very short /m/, produce it quickly with tension, and then explode it. You may need to instruct the client to pinch his nose shut while producing the /m/ so to force the air out through the mouth, resulting in a /b/.

4. Shape /b/ from /hu/. Tell the client to sustain /hu/ and then slowly bring the lips together. This is recommended to elicit voicing when /p/ is substantiated for /b/. The syllable /hju/ is also suggested as a point of departure.

5. Shape /b/ from /u/. Tell the client to sustain /u/ with the lips pursed and as close to touching as possible. Then run your forefinger rapidly across the lips. This should produce a sequence resembling /bu, bu, bu, bu/.

/t/

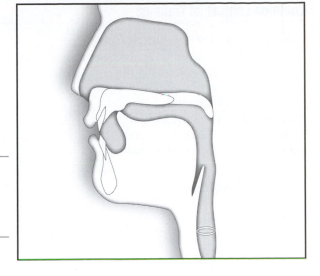

PMV Features:

Lingua (Apical -*tip*)
alveolar/stop/voiceless

Production:

The tongue apex is raised
to contact the alveolar
ridge while the sides of the tongue contact the upper teeth (molars and gums),
forming a seal. The tongue tip is suddenly pulled away from the alveolar ridge
to release the unvoiced intra-oral breath pressure in the form of a sudden aspi-
rate (breathy) burst of energy.

Common Errors:

1. Voicing: d/t

2. Dorsal-velar: k/t

3. Laminal-alveolar/fricative: s/t

4. Apical-dental/fricative: θ/t

5. Imprecise /t/

    a. Laminal-alveolar placement
    b. Dental placement

6. Cosmetic /t/; acoustically correct but incorrect placement

7. Air wastage by nasal emission

8. Omission

Common Contextual Variants:

Unrounded /t/: tea, tip, tack, tub
Rounded /tʷ/: tune, tool, toe, took
Unaspirated /t⁼/: stick, stay, stool
No audible release burst /t̚/: utmost
Dental /t̪/: tenth, eighth
Nasal release /tⁿ/: satin, button
Lateral release /tˡ/: settle, metal, kettle
Flap/tap /ɾ/: writer, butter, matter, data

Eliciting Techniques:

Phonetic Placement

Demonstrate the feature characteristics of /t/:

- Tongue tip to alveolar ridge

- Explosion of air (breathy)

- Velum closed

- Vocal folds silent

1. Tell the client to hold the tongue firmly against the alveolar ridge (a mirror could be used here to show the client the correct placement). Then have him quickly lower his tongue. This may produce an approximation of /t/ (Bernthal and Bankson, 1981). The result is a production that is almost right so the clinician may only need to "fine tune" it by gradually shaping the amount of air released and the rapid movement needed for correct production. It is usually good to signal the proper movement with your fingertip to demonstrate its force and rapidity.

2. Show the amount of pressure of the tongue necessary to produce /t/. Use a tongue depressor or the client's finger pressed on the client's tongue tip.

3. Demonstrate by analogy the sudden release of the tongue by pressing the client's hands together and then suddenly separating them.

4. Show the plosive release necessary for /t/. Demonstrate the plosive burst on the back of the client's hand. Have the client then attempt to do the same thing on his hand.

5. Hold a piece of string, a feather, or a lightweight paper in front of your mouth to demonstrate explosive release. Instruct the client to place his tongue directly behind his upper central incisors against the alveolar ridge. Tell the client to blow out through his mouth while lowering his tongue. Draw attention to the movement of the string, feather, or paper.

6. Touch the alveolar ridge with the end of a tongue depressor. Instruct the client to touch the bump just behind the central incisors (front two teeth). Ask the client to place the tip of his tongue there to begin the sound.

7. To emphasize the placement of the tongue, wet the end of a cotton swab and rub it on a flavored food, such as a mint Lifesaver. Touch the client's alveolar ridge with the swab to teach correct placement. Some clinicians use peanut butter (be cautious about food allergies). Ask the client to remove the food with the tongue tip as he feels the bump behind his central incisors (which for younger children can be referred to as the "magic spot"). Then instruct the client to place the tongue tip on the alveolar ridge (magic spot), then release the tongue while blowing air out of the mouth.

8. Hold the client's lower jaw down slightly. Have the client practice raising and lowering the tongue tip to the alveolar ridge.

9. Instruct the client to rest the underside of his tongue on the end of a tongue depressor. Tell him to keep the tongue on the tongue depressor (the "shelf," according to Bleile, 2004). Using the "shelf," guide the tongue up to the alveolar ridge and back down again to show the correct placement and suggest the proper movement. As a variation, use a piece of gauze and actually manipulate the client's tongue tip held between your thumb and forefinger. Then, instruct the client to touch "the bump" behind his upper central incisors (front two teeth) quickly with his tongue tip.

10. Use hand gestures to demonstrate how to tap the tongue against the alveolar ridge.

11. Hold a tongue depressor vertically so that the top edge rests on the alveolar ridge. Tell the client to explode air with the tip of his tongue directly at the tongue depressor.

12. As a touch cue, lay your finger above the top lip.

13. Remind the client of the dripping sound, the popping sound, the tapping sound, the tongue tapper or the "quiet brother" sound (Lindamood and Lindamood, 1998), as well as the tippy sound, bump sound, and hill sound.

14. It can also be called the short sound, or tick-tock sound.

Moto-Kinesthetic

With your forefinger, touch the middle area just above the client's upper lip. Using only a small amount of pressure (stimulation with your finger), move your forefinger in a downward stroke to suggest the appropriate tongue movement.

Sound Approximation

1. Instruct the client to make a /p/ + schwa. Ask him to place the tongue tip between the lips and say /p/ + schwa. Then, instruct him to make a similar sound with the tongue tip contacting the upper lip. Finally, have him try it by touching the alveolar ridge behind the upper front teeth.

2. Shape /t/ from /l/. Instruct the client to produce a hard, whispered /l/ sound. Then, tell him to produce several of these sounds.

3. Shape /t/ from /l/. Ask the client to say a series of sounds that begin with /h/ and end quickly in a whispered /l/.

4. Shape /t/ from /d/. Ask the client to say /d/ several times. Then, tell him to whisper the /d/. Having him feel this throat with his hand to sense voice versus voiceless will also help. An alternative direction is to tell the client to "turn off the motor, buzzing sound or voice box."

5. Shape /t/ from /tʃ/. Ask him to say /tʃ/ while you hold your hands on his lips to inhibit pursing.

6. Tell the client to say /d/ while turning off the voicing (i.e., "turning off the voice box, turning off the motor sound or turning off the buzzing sound").

/d/

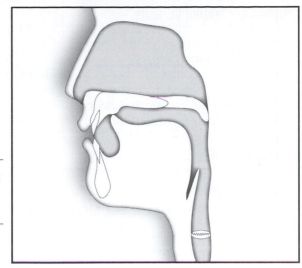

PMV Features:

Apical-alveolar/stop/voiced

Production:

As the voiced cognate of /t/, /d/ is produced similarly. The tongue apex is raised to contact the alveolar ridge while the sides of the tongue contact the upper teeth (molars and gums), forming a seal. Voicing begins, and then the tongue tip is suddenly pulled away from the alveolar ridge to release the intra-oral breath pressure in the form of a suddenburst of energy that is less aspirated (breathy) and less tense than /t/.

Common Errors:

1. Devoicing: t/d
2. Dorsal-velar: g/d
3. Apical-dental/fricative: ð/d
4. Laminal-alveolar/fricative: z/d
5. Imprecise /d/:
   - laminal-alveolar placement
   - dental placement
6. Cosmetic /d/; acoustically correct but incorrect placement
7. Air wastage by nasal emission
8. Omission

Common Contextual Variants:

Unrounded /d/: dean, dip, date, dub
Rounded /dʷ/: dune, dote, dude
No audible release burst /dˀ/: bedroom, madman, beds
Nasal release /dⁿ/: sadden, leaden
Lateral release /dᴸ/: bundle, handle, paddle
Flap/tap /ɾ/: seeding, leader, fading

Eliciting Techniques:

Phonetic Placement

The principles involved in eliciting /d/ are essentially similar to /t/. Demonstrate the feature characteristics of /d/:

- Tongue tip to alveolar ridge

- *Slight* explosion of air

- Velum closed

- Vocal folds vibrating

1. Tell the client to hold the tongue firmly against the alveolar ridge (a mirror could be used here to show the client the correct placement). Then, have him quickly lower his tongue. This may produce an approximation of /d/. The result is a production that is almost right so the clinician may only need to "fine tune" it by gradually shaping the amount of air released and the rapid movement needed for correct production of /d/. Again, as with /t/, it is usually useful to signal the proper movement with your fingertip to demonstrate its force and rapidity.

2. Show the amount of pressure exerted by the tip of the tongue by touching the client's tongue tip with a tongue depressor.

3. Demonstrate by analogy the sudden release of the tongue by pressing the client's hands together and then suddenly separating them.

4. Hold a piece of string, feather, or lightweight paper in front of your mouth to demonstrate explosive release. Instruct the client to place his tongue directly behind his upper central incisors against the alveolar ridge. Tell the client to blow out through his mouth while lowering his tongue. Draw attention to the movement of the string, feather, or paper.

5. Touch the alveolar ridge with the end of a tongue depressor. Instruct the client to touch bump just behind the lateral incisors (front two teeth). Ask the client to place the tip of his tongue there to begin the sound.

6. To emphasize the placement of the tongue, wet the end of a cotton swab and rub it on a flavored food, such as a Lifesaver. Touch the client's alveolar ridge with the swab to teach correct placement. Some clinicians use peanut butter (be cautious about food allergies). Ask the client to remove the food with the tongue tip as he feels the bump behind his central incisors (which for younger children can be referred to as the "magic spot"). Now, instruct the client to place the tongue tip on the alveolar ridge (magic spot), then release the tongue while blowing air out of the mouth.

7. Hold the client's lower jaw down slightly. Have the client practice raising and lowering the tongue tip to the alveolar ridge.

8. Instruct the client to rest the underside of his tongue on the end of a tongue depressor. Tell him to keep the tongue on the tongue depressor (the "shelf," according to Bleile, 2004). Using the "shelf," guide the tongue up to the alveolar ridge and down again to show the correct placement and movement. As a variation, to use a piece of gauze and actually manipulate the client's tongue tip between your thumb and forefinger. Then, instruct the client to touch "the bump" behind his upper central incisors (front two teeth) quickly with his tongue tip.

9. Hold a tongue depressor vertically so the top edge rests on the alveolar ridge. Tell the client to explode air with the tip of his tongue directly at the tongue depressor. It is important to demonstrate the voicing before the closure release. Remind young children that "the motor comes on first."

10. Contrast the plosive release for /t/ and /d/ (with the /d/ being less forceful in the degree of burst of air and the tension) on the back of the client's hand. As with /t/, this may also be done with a thin strip of lightweight paper. First, demonstrate /t/ and /d/, and then let the client attempt it.

11. Contrast voicing differences between /t/ and /d/. Instruct the client to hold his hand lightly on your throat as you produce each sound. Then have him do the same on himself. For the younger child, refer to the voiced component by saying "use the buzzing sound" or "turn on your motor." Again, it is important that voicing is demonstrated before the closure release.

12. As a touch cue, lay your finger above the top lip.

13. Remind the client to think of the dripping sound, the popping sound, the tapping sound, the tongue tapper sound, or the "noisy brother" of /t/ (Lindamood and Lindamood, 1998), as well as the tippy sound, the bump sound, the hill sound, the short sound, the "do" sound, the woodpecker sound, or the jackhammer sound.

Moto-Kinesthetic

The stimulation for /d/ is the same as that for /t/, except a little more forefinger pressure is applied to suggest voicing.

Sound Approximation

1. Instruct the client to make a /b/ + schwa. Then ask him to place the tongue tip between the lips and again try to say /b/ + schwa. Then instruct him to make a similar sound (a sound almost like the /b/ sound) with the tongue tip contacting the upper lip. Finally, have him try placing the tongue tip on the alveolar ridge behind the upper front teeth.

2. Shape /d/ from /l/. Tell the client to put his tongue where he makes /l/. Then tell him to press hard and explode some air.

3. Shape /d/ from /ð/. Have the client progressively approximate explosive productions of /ðə/. The principle here is to begin by saying exploded (rapid) productions of *the* and gradually retracting the tongue to the alveolar ridge.

4. Shape /d/ from /ʌ/. Instruct the client to prolong /ʌ/ and stop that with his tongue tip quickly to the alveolar ridge. Then have him say a series of these sounds. What may result is /ʌd, ʌd, də, də/.

5. Tell the client to say /t/ while turning on the voicing (i.e., turning on the voice box, turning on the motor sound or turning on the buzzing sound).

/k/

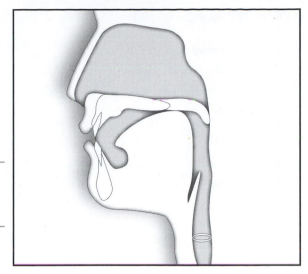

PMV Features:

Dorsal-velar/stop/voiceless

Production:

The dorsum of the tongue is raised to contact the soft palate, second molars, and posterior gum ridge to form a seal, which completely blocks the airstream. The back of the tongue is suddenly pulled away from the velum to release unvoiced intra-oral breath pressure in the form of a sudden aspirated (breathy) burst of energy.

Common Errors:

1. Apical-alveolar: t/k
2. Glottal/fricative: h/k
3. Voicing: g/k
4. Excessive or insufficient pressure release, i.e., substitution of post-dorsal-velar fricative
5. Gutteral /k/ (post-dorsal-uvular stop)
6. Omission

Common Contextual Variants:

Advanced /k̟/: key, cute, kit
Retracted /k̠/: cool, cot, could
Unrounded /k/: tea, tip, tack, tub
Rounded /kʷ/: cool, coal, coat, cook
Unaspirated /k˭/: ski, sky, scan
No audible release burst /k̚/: luckless

Eliciting Techniques:

Phonetic Placement

Demonstrate the feature charact eristics of /k/:

- Back (dorsum) of tongue raised to soft palate (velar placement)
- Explosion of air (breathy)
- Velum closed
- Vocal folds silent

1. Demonstrate the plosive release of /k/ on the back side of your hand and then on the client's hand.

2. To demonstrate by analogy the sudden release of the tongue, press the client's hands together and then suddenly separate them.

3. Hold a piece of string, a feather, or a lightweight paper in front of your mouth to demonstrate explosive release. Draw attention to the movement of the string, feather, or paper.

4. Because so little of the tongue movement for /k/ is visible, illustrations of tongue placement (drawings, diagrams, or hand gesture to show the scraping of the tongue against the roof of the mouth) are helpful. To emphasize the velar placement, have the client cough or gargle.

5. Place the client's hands on your uppermost part of the neck under the client's jaw near the throat. You produce the /k/. Then draw attention to the muscle movement to point out the velar placement.

6. Use a tongue depressor to guide the tongue toward a backward movement.

7. Ask the client to feel your throat when you say /k/ to illustrate devoicing and motion in the back of the mouth.

8. Have the client look in the mirror as you demonstrate the position of the tongue tip behind the lower incisors

9. Tell the client to anchor the tongue against the lower teeth and hold his hand in the front of his mouth to feel the burst of air while he imitates your production (Van Riper, 1963).

10. Press underneath the back of the client's chin and tell him to whisper /k/ in an explosive manner (Van Riper, 1963).

11. Using a tongue depressor, hold the tongue tip down behind the lower teeth to hinder the elevation of the tongue tip. Tell the client to make his tongue hump up in the back and force air at that spot. Then direct him to explode that air quickly (Bernthal and Bankson, 1981).

12. Rub a moist cotton swab on a flavored food, such as a Lifesaver. Peanut butter is good alternative; yet be cautious about food allergies. Then touch the soft

palate near the second molars with the swab and ask the client to raise the back of the tongue to the roof of the mouth to form a seal. Finally, instruct him to release the back of the tongue quickly so to create a burst of air.

13. Instruct the client to make the /g/ sound and then turn off the voice box, the buzzing sound, or the motor.

14. As a touch cue, lay your fingers on the uppermost part of the client's neck.

15. Refer to the /k/ as the throaty sound, the back sound, the short sound, the dripping sound, the coughing sound, the cawing-crow sound, the tongue-scraper sound, or the "quiet brother" of /g/ (Lindamood and Lindamood, 1998).

Moto-Kinesthetic

Using latex gloves, the clinician places her thumb and forefinger under the client's jaw near the throat, the thumb on one side of the throat, the forefinger on the other side. She applies pressure upward and downward to suggest the lifting and releasing of the back of the tongue.

Sound Approximation

1. Have the client say /t/. The /t/ can be used to illustrate the build up of pressure and the quick release. Then have him attempt saying /t/ with the tongue tip behind the lower central incisors. Follow with the step of instructing the client to raise the back of the tongue up to the soft palate and attempt the /k/ production.

2. Direct the client to say /i/. While sustaining the /i/, the client should then raise the back of the tongue to touch the soft palate near the second molars. Once the contact is made and a seal is formed, tell the client to release the tongue quickly.

3. Have the client practice saying *puh-tuh-kuh* slowly, then increase the speed.

4. Shape /k/ from /ŋ/. Instruct the client to lightly explode air in the quiet production of /ŋ/.

5. Tell the client to cough or imitate a cough.

6. Have the client practice front-back movements of /t/ and /k/.

7. Shape /k/ from /g/. Ask the client to whisper a /gə/.

8. To eliminate a gutteral /k/ posturing, have the client repeat /i/-/k/ in rapid sequence, trying to keep the tongue in the /k/ posture while saying the /i/.

9. Tell the client to swallow at the same time he attempts /k/.

10. Tell the client to prolong /h/ and then cough; or tell him to swallow while exploding the air of /h/.

/g/

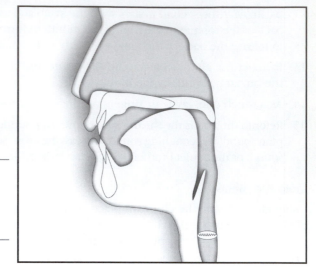

PMV Features:

Dorsal (back)
velar/stop/voiced

Production:

As the voiced cognate of
/k/, /g/ is produced simi-
larly. The dorsum of the tongue is raised to contact the velum, second molars,
and the posterior gum ridge forming a seal which completely blocks the airstream. Voicing begins, and then the back of the tongue is suddenly pulled
away from the velum to release intra-oral breath pressure in the form of a sudden burst of energy, less aspirated (breathy), and with less tension than /k/.

Common Errors:

1. Apical-alveolar: d/g
2. (Gutteral) glottal/fricative: h/k
3. Devoicing: k/g
4. Excess or insufficient pressure release, i.e., substitution of a post-dorsal
   velar fricative
5. Omission

Common Contextual Variants:

Advanced /g̟/: give, get, gill
Retracted /g̠/: good, got, goo, ghoul
Unrounded /g/: God, gate, guy
Rounded /gʷ/: go, ghoul, good
No audible release burst /g̚/: ugly, mugs, lugnut

Eliciting Techniques:

Phonetic Placement

The principles involved in eliciting /g/ are essentially similar to those for /k/; simply instruct the client to add the voicing feature. Demonstrate feature characteristics of /g/:

- Back (dorsum) of the tongue contacting the velum (velar placement)
- Slight explosion of air
- Velum closed
- Vocal folds vibrating

1. Demonstrate the plosive release of /g/ on the back side of your hand and then on the client's hand.

2. To demonstrate by analogy the sudden release of the tongue, press the client's hands together and then suddenly separate them. It is important to demonstrate the voicing before the closure release. Remind young children that "the motor comes on first."

3. Hold a piece of string, a feather, or a lightweight paper in front of your mouth to demonstrate explosive release. Draw attention to the movement of the string, feather, or paper.

4. Because so little of the tongue movement for /g/ is visible, illustrations of tongue placement (drawings, diagrams, or hand gestures to show the scraping of the tongue against the roof of the mouth) are helpful. To emphasize the velar placement, have the client cough or gargle.

5. Place the client's hands on your uppermost part of the neck on the under the client's jaw near the throat. You produce the /g/. Then draw attention to the muscle movement to point out the velar placement.

6. Use a tongue depressor to guide the tongue in a backward movement.

7. Ask the client to feel your throat when you say /g/ to illustrate voicing and motion in the back of the mouth.

8. Have the client look in the mirror as you demonstrate the position of the tongue tip behind the lower incisors.

9. Tell the client to anchor the tongue against the lower teeth and hold his hand in the front of his mouth to feel the burst of air while he imitates your production (Van Riper, 1963).

10. Press underneath the back of the client's chin and tell him to whisper /g/ in an explosive manner (Van Riper, 1963).

11. Hold the tongue tip down behind the lower teeth with a tongue depressor to hinder the elevation of the tongue tip. Tell the client to make his tongue hump up in the back and force air at that spot. Then direct him to explode that air quickly (Bernthal and Bankson, 1981).

12. Rub a moist cotton swab on a flavored food, such as a mint Lifesaver. Peanut butter is good alternative; yet be cautious about food allergies. Then touch the soft palate near the second molars with the swab and ask the client to raise the back of the tongue to the roof of the mouth to form a seal. Then instruct him release the back of the tongue quickly so to create a burst of air.

13. Instruct the client to make the /k/ sound and then turn on the voice box, the buzzing sound, or the motor.

14. As a touch cue, lay your fingers on the uppermost part of the client's neck.

15. Refer to the /g/ as the throaty sound, the back sound, the short sound, the dripping sound, the coughing sound, the water-pouring sound (glug, glug), the frog sound, the baby-babbling sound, the tongue-scraper sound, or the "noisy brother" of /k/ (Lindamood and Lindamood, 1998).

Moto-Kinesthetic

The moto-kinesthetic stimulation for /g/ is similar to that for /k/ except more pressure is used as you press upward and inward and then release pressure. You do not stimulate any downward action as you did for /k/. The suggestion for voicing is also made.

Sound Approximation

1. Have the client say /d/. The /d/ can be used to illustrate the build-up of pressure and the quick release. Have him attempt saying /t/ with the tongue tip behind the lower central incisors. Then instruct the client to raise the back of the tongue up to the soft palate and attempt to produce /g/.

2. Direct the client to say and sustain /i/. Then instruct him to raise the back of the tongue to touch the soft palate near the second molars. Once the contact is made and a seal is formed, tell the client to release the tongue quickly.

3. Tell the client to practice saying *buh-duh-guh* slowly and then increase the speed.

4. Shape /g/ from /ŋ/. Tell the client to forcefully explode /ŋ/.

5. Tell the client to cough or imitate a cough while holding one hand on his throat. Instruct him to voice that coughing sound.

6. Practice front-back movements of /d/ and /g/.

7. Shape /g/ from /k/. Have the client hold one hand on his throat and voice the /k/ sound.

8. Tell the client to swallow while attempting /g/.

9. Instruct the client to hold his thumb and forefinger under his chin in the same manner you did in the moto-kinesthetic stimulation. Then have him prolong /ʌ/ and arrest it by pressing inward and upward as he attempts /g/. A favorable result resembles /ʌ . . . gə/.

/s/

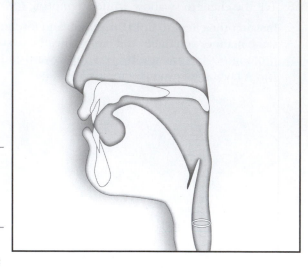

PMV Features:

Lingua (laminal) alveolar/
fricative/voiceless

Production:

The blade of the tongue is
raised to nearly contact the
alveolar ridge, while the sides (lateral edges) of the tongue contact the upper
teeth. This creates a small groove at the midline of the tongue. The unvoiced
airstream is then directed through this constriction producing a noisy friction-
like sound.

Additional information on /s/ is presented in Appendix C, where Dr.
Richard Shine discusses three types of lisping behaviors and presents an
elicitation procedure he has used successfully with clients for several years.
Although Shine's procedure can be used with all types of lisps, it is especially
effective in the treatment of the lateral /s/ lisp.

Common Errors:

1. Apical-dental: θ/s
2. Laminal-prepalatal: ʃ/s
3. Glottal: h/s
4. Labiodental: f/s
5. Voicing: z/s
6. Apical-alveolar/affricate: ts/s
7. Apical-alveolar/stop: t/s
8. Palato–alveolar/affricate: tʃ/s
9. Apical-alveolar/stop/voiced: d/s
10. Lateral emission: lateral /s/
11. Insufficient breath pressure

12. Whistling /s/

13. Nasal emission

14. Omission

Common Contextual Variants:

Unrounded /s/: seat, sip, say, sad
Rounded /sʷ/: soon, so, soap, suit
Dental /s̪/: tenths

Eliciting Techniques:

Phonetic Placement

Demonstrate the feature characteristics of /s/:

- Blade of the tongue nearly touching the alveolar ridge
- Lateral edges raised to contact the inner surfaces of the upper back teeth
- Slow release of air over the tongue toward the cutting edges of upper central incisors
- Velum closed
- Vocal folds silent

Note: Techniques followed by a double asterisk (**) are especially good for lateral /s/.

1. Demonstrate this procedure step-by-step in a mirror first, and then allow the client to attempt the same:
    a. Raise the back of the tongue so he can feel his upper back teeth.
    b. Place the tip of the tongue behind his upper front teeth and then pull it away from them slightly.
    c. Close his teeth so that they are barely touching.
    d. The clinician should then hold the tip of her finger in front of the center of the client's mouth and say, "Blow air slowly over your tongue toward my finger."

2. For /s/ with the tongue tip down:
    a. Position the back of the tongue to contact the upper back teeth.
    b. Place the tongue tip behind lower central incisors (you may need a tongue depressor).
    c. Close the teeth.
    d. Initiate /s/.

3. To develop a central airstream, use any of these techniques:

   a.   Draw a small target and hold it in front of the mouth. Tell the client to make a bull's-eye with the /s/.

   b.   Hold your fingertip about three inches from the client's nose. Ask him to force the /s/ outward and upward toward your finger, or have the client use his own finger.

   c.   Have the client close his teeth and direct the airstream for /s/ through a straw.

   d.   Use a tongue depressor and trace a line through the center of his tongue to give the client the idea of a trough before attempting /s/.

   e.   Tell the client to pucker his lips and then fully retract them. Push the tongue forward and say /s/.

   f.   Place the client's finger at the very center of the teeth and have him attempt /s/.

4. Use a tongue depressor to show precise points of contact in the mouth. Then place the edge of the tongue depressor just behind the teeth (either the upper or lower incisors). Ask the client to hold it there with his tongue tip. The small opening created when you remove the tongue depressor is almost the distance necessary for air to pass in order to secure /s/. Ask the client to blow air outwardly, resulting in the /s/.

5. Instruct the client to close his teeth and rapidly bring the back of the tongue up against the upper teeth while attempting /s/.

6. Tell the client to groove the tongue and then attempt /s/.

7. Instruct him to close his teeth and bring his lips together tightly. Then slowly open the lips to allow the /s/ to escape.

8. Instruct the client to make a little smile and to hide his tongue behind the "white gate" (his teeth), while resting the sides of his tongue along his upper back teeth. Tell the client to blow straight out with a fine stream of air. Using your index finger to indicate the central emission of the airstream may be helpful.

9. Tell the client to bite down slightly on the back teeth. Use your index finger and thumb to touch the outside of the cheeks at the location of the juncture of the upper first and second molars. Then tell the client to blow the air straight out the front of his mouth. Use your index finger to show the pathway straight out from the lips to indicate the emission of the central airstream.**

10. Use a tongue depressor to make a "shelf" for the tongue to rest on. Place the tongue depressor against the lower edges of the upper incisors. Instruct the client to place the tongue on the "shelf," and raise the tongue up behind the upper front teeth. If needed, use the tongue depressor to lift the tongue. Direct the client to contact the lateral edges of the tongue with the back teeth and blow out.

11. As a touch cue, point to the corners of the mouth to encourage spreading of the lips, and then remind the client to put his teeth together.

12. Remind the client to use the snake sound, the whistling tea kettle sound, the hissing sound, the bump sound, the hill sound, the skinny air sound, or the "quiet brother" of /z/ (Lindamood and Lindamood, 1998).

Moto-Kinesthetic

Using latex gloves, place the thumb and forefinger of your left hand at the corners of the client's upper lip. Place the thumb and forefinger of your right hand on the corners of the lower lip. If the occlusion is normal, push the lower jaw into the position of a normal bite; then pull the lower jaw down to create a very slight opening between the teeth. Ask the client to blow air through the teeth.

Sound Approximation

1. Instruct the client to bring the teeth together and "slurp" inhaled air. Then he should exhale this air as /s/.

2. Shape /s/ from /θ/. Instruct the client to prolong /θ/ as in *think*. Tell him to gradually bring his tongue into the mouth over the back of the top front teeth and along the alveolar ridge to the vicinity for /s/ while saying /θ/. Incorporate these variations:

   a. Use a tongue depressor to guide the movement.
   b. Use the tongue tip to "point" the back of the teeth and the gum ridge.
   c. Tell the client to say a list of initial position /θ/ words slowly. As he utters the /θ/ sound in each word, push the tongue inward and upward to the alveolar area with a tongue depressor.

3. Shape /s/ from /t/. Instruct the client to make rapid productions of /t/ and prolong the last one into /s/.

   A variation of this technique is to shape the /s/ from a /ts/ context, such as in the word *boat* (i.e., "boat → boats"). Have the client focus on how the /t/ feels and hold it while producing the /s/. You may need to prompt the client to drop the tongue. Bernthal and Bankson (2004) suggest "sneaking up quietly" on the /s/ while deleting the /t/. **

4. Shape /s/ from /[tʰ]. Tell the client to say /t/ with a great amount of plosion. This considerably aspirated /t/ will result in the German affricate /ts/. Ask the client to prolong the second sound in /ts/ (e.g., /ts/ – /ts/ = tssssss).

5. Shape /s/ from /i/. Instruct the client to say /i/ and then gradually close the teeth and say /s/ while turning off the voicing (voice box).

6. Shape /s/ from /ʃ/. Tell the client to say /ʃ/, smile, and push the tongue slightly forward.

7. Shape /s/ from /z/. Tell the client to whisper a /z/, or have him hold his hand on his throat while he produces /z/ and then turns off the voicing.

8. Shape /s/ from /n/. Tell the client to place his tongue where he says /n/ and then to release the tongue slightly and force air over the tongue.

9. Shape /s/ from /l/. Tell the client to put his tongue up for /l/, close his teeth, and release his tongue slightly, then blow air over his tongue.

10. Shape /s/ from /h/. Instruct the client to close his teeth, then prolong /h/ while he gradually raises the tongue tip.

11. Shape /s/ from /f/. Instruct the client to lift the tongue tip slowly as he prolongs /f/ and slowly brings his front teeth together.

/z/

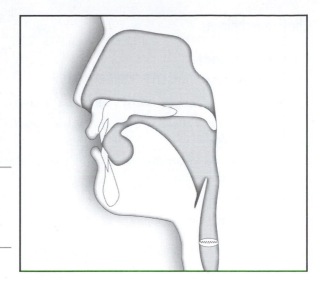

PMV Features:

Lingua-laminal) alveolar/
fricative/voiced

Production:

As the voiced cognate of
/s/, /z/ is produced simi-
larly. The blade of the tongue is raised to nearly contact the alveolar ridge, while
the sides (lateral edges) of the tongue contact the upper teeth. This creates a
small groove at the midline of the tongue. The voiced airstream is then directed
through this constriction, producing friction, although with less tension than /s/.

Common Errors:

1. Apical-dental: ð/z
2. Apical-dental unvoiced: θ/z
3. Palato-alveolar: ʒ/z
4. Labiodental: v/z
5. Apical-alveolar/stop: d/z
6. Apical-alveolar/stop/unvoiced: t/z
7. Glottal/unvoiced: h/z
8. Unvoiced: h/z
9. Lateral emission: lateral /z/
10. No aperture for emission of /z/
11. Omission

Common Contextual Variants:

Unrounded /z/: zip, zap, zero
Rounded /zʷ/: zone, zoo, zoom
Dental /z̪/: bathes

Eliciting Techniques:

Phonetic Placement

Demonstrate the feature characteristics of /z/:

- Blade of the tongue nearly touching the alveolar ridge
- Lateral edges raised to contact the inner surfaces of the upper back teeth
- Slow release of air over the tongue toward the cutting edges of upper central incisors
- Velum closed
- Vocal folds vibrating

Note: Techniques followed by a double asterisk (**) are especially good for lateral /z/.

1. Demonstrate this procedure step-by-step in a mirror, and then allow the client to attempt the same:

   a. Raise the back of the tongue so he can feel his upper back teeth.
   b. Place the tip of the tongue behind his upper front teeth and then pull it away slightly from them.
   c. Close his teeth so that they are barely touching.
   d. The clinician should then hold the tip of her finger in front of the center of the client's mouth and say, "Blow air slowly over your tongue toward my finger, and make your vocal cords go at the same time."

2. For /z/ with the tongue tip down:

   a. Place the back of the tongue next to upper back teeth.
   b. Place the tongue tip behind lower central incisors (you may need a tongue depressor for this).
   c. Close the teeth.
   d. Initiate /z/.

3. To develop a central airstream, use any of these techniques:

   a. Draw a small target and hold it in front of the mouth. Tell the client to make a bull's-eye with the /z/.
   b. Hold your fingertip just above the client's upper lip. Ask him to force the /z/ outward and upward toward your finger; or have the client use his own finger.
   c. Have the client close his teeth and direct the airstream for /z/ through a straw.
   d. Using a tongue depressor, trace a line through the center of his tongue to give the client the idea of a trough.

    e.   Tell the client to pucker his lips, then fully retract them, push the tongue forward, and say /z/.

    f.   Place the client's finger at the very center of the teeth and have him attempt /z/.

4. Use a tongue depressor to show precise points of contact in the mouth. Then place the edge of the tongue depressor just behind the teeth (either the upper or lower incisors). Ask the client to hold it there with his tongue tip. The small opening created when you remove the tongue depressor is almost the distance necessary for air to pass in order to secure /z/. Make sure the client holds one hand on his throat to feel the vocal folds vibrating.

5. Instruct the client to close the teeth and rapidly bring the back of the tongue up against the upper teeth while attempting /z/.

6. Tell the client to groove the tongue and then attempt /z/.

7. Instruct him to close his teeth and bring his lips together tightly. Then slowly open the lips to allow the /z/ to escape.

8. Instruct the client to make a little smile and to hide his tongue behind the "white gate" (his teeth), while resting the sides of his tongue along his upper back teeth and blowing straight out with a fine stream of air. Using your index finger to indicate the central emission of the airstream may be helpful. Remind the client to turn on his voice box.

9. Tell the client to bite down slightly on his back teeth (using your index finger and thumb to touch the outside of the cheeks at the location of the juncture of the upper first and second molars), and blow the air straight out the front of his mouth. Indicate the emission of the central airstream by using your index finger to show the pathway straight out from the lips. Instruct the client to make sure the sound is voiced; instruct the younger child to turn on his motor as you touch his laryngeal area.

10. Use a tongue depressor to make a "shelf" for the tongue to rest on. Place the tongue depressor against the lower edges of the upper incisors. Instruct the client to place his tongue on the "shelf," and raise the tongue up behind the upper front teeth. If necessary, use the tongue depressor to lift the tongue. Direct the client to contact the lateral edges of the tongue with the back teeth and breathe out he voices the production of the target /z/.

11. As a touch cue, point to the corners of the mouth to encourage spreading of the lips, and then remind the client to put his teeth together.

12. Remind the client to use the bee sound, the hissing sound, the bump sound, the hill sound, the skinny air sound, or the "noisy brother" of /s/ (Lindamood and Lindamood, 1998).

Moto-Kinesthetic

Using latex gloves, place the thumb and forefinger of your left hand at the corners of the client's upper lip. Place the thumb and forefinger of your right hand on the corners of the lower lip. If the occlusion is normal, push the lower jaw into the position of a normal bite; then pull the lower jaw down to create a slight opening between the teeth. Ask the client to blow air through the teeth. To suggest voicing, place the client's hand on his throat.

Sound Approximation

1. Instruct the client to bring his teeth together and "slurp" inhaled air, then he should exhale this air as /z/. **

2. Shape /z/ from /ð/. Instruct the client to prolong /ð/ as in *them*. Tell him to gradually bring the tongue into the mouth over the back of the top teeth and along the alveolar ridge to the vicinity for /z/ while saying /ð/. Incorporate these variations:

   a. Use a tongue depressor to guide the movement.
   b. Use the tongue tip to "point" the back of the teeth and the gum ridge.
   c. Tell the client to say a list of initial position /ð/ words slowly (e.g., these, those, they). As he utters the /ð/ sound in each word, push the tongue inward and upward to the alveolar area with a tongue depressor.

3. Shape /z/ from /d/. Instruct the client to make rapid productions of /d/ and prolong the last one into /z/. **

4. Shape /z/ from /d/. Tell the client to say /d/ very fast, almost like a trilling of /d/. This will produce something like /dz/. Ask the client to prolong the second sound in /dz/ (e.g., /dz-dz-dzzzzzz/). **

5. Shape /z/ from /i/. Instruct the client to say /i/, then to gradually close the teeth and say /z/.

6. Shape /z/ from /ʒ/. Tell the client to say /ʒ/, and then to smile and push the tongue slightly forward.

7. Shape /z/ from /s/. Tell the client to prolong /s/. Have him hold one hand on his throat while he produces /s/. Then instruct him to turn voicing on.

8. Shape /z/ from /n/. Tell the client to place his tongue where he says /n/. Then he should release the tongue slightly and force air over the tongue while he produces voice.

9. Shape /z/ from /l/. Tell the client to put his tongue up for /l/, close his teeth and release his tongue slightly, and then blow air over the tongue while he produces voice.

10. Shape /z/ from /hi/. Instruct the client to close his teeth, then prolong /hi/ while he gradually raises his tongue.

11. Shape /z/ from /v/. Instruct the client to lift the tongue tip slowly as he prolongs /v/ and gracefully brings his front teeth together.

/f/

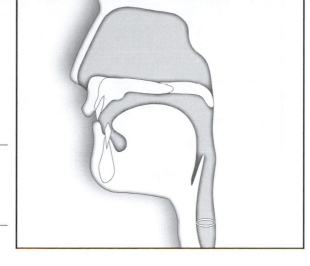

PMV Features:

Labiodental/fricative/
voiceless

Production:

The lower edges of the
upper teeth are brought
into contact with the lower lip to create a constriction in the oral cavity. The
mandible tends to close, which aids the lower lip in constricting the airstream.
The unvoiced airstream is then directed through this constriction to produce
friction.

Common Errors:

1. Apical-dental: θ/f
2. Bilabial/stop: p/f
3. Bilabial/stop/voicing: b/f
4. Laminal-alveolar: s/f
5. Voicing: v/f
6. Insufficient or excess air pressure
7. Voiceless bilabial fricative (the gesture of blowing out a candle): φ/f
8. Omission

Common Contextual Variants:

Unrounded /f/: feel, fit, fat, fake
Rounded /f^w/: fool, full, foal, food

Eliciting Techniques:

Phonetic Placement

Demonstrate the feature characteristics of /f/:

- Lower edges of upper teeth lightly contacting the lower lip
- Air passing through the small teeth-lip opening
- Velum closed
- Vocal folds silent

1. Instruct the client to place his upper teeth on his lower lip and blow air over his lip.

2. Tell the client to make a small smile and bite down lightly on his lower lip with his upper teeth. Hold a strip of lightweight paper in front of his mouth and tell him to blow air lightly. Use a tongue depressor to elicit the proper shape of the lips and the appropriate opening for the air to pass through.

3. Show the client the exact articulatory position of /f/ in a mirror. Tell him not to bite on his lip, but to open them a little bit and lightly blow air. Instruct the client to lick his lower lip and then to repeat the /f/ production, drawing attention to the air as it "cools" the lower lip. Label /f/ the Lip Cooler to associate the cooling off of the lip with the sound production (Lindamood and Lindamood, 1998).

4. Instruct the client to close his mouth so that the lower lip barely touches the upper teeth. Next, hold the client's finger crosswise between the lips and ask the client to blow air, which will result in the /f/ sound.

5. Practice different labiodental positions. Ask the client to position his upper teeth far down over the lower lip. Have him blow air and gradually move the cutting edges of his upper teeth into the appropriate /f/ placement.

6. Instruct the client to pucker and blow air while he slowly changes the shape of the lips into a smile.

7. Tell the client to make a "jack-o-lantern" face (Flowers, 1980) while smiling and touching the upper teeth to the lower lips. Position a strip of lightweight paper in front of the client's mouth, and instruct the client to blow out to move it to draw attention to the direction and force of the airstream.

8. Place a small piece of hypo-allergenic tape on the lower lip to develop an awareness of the use of the lower lip

9. As a touch cue, lay the client's finger below his bottom lip.

10. Tell the client to use the angry cat sound, the biting lip sound, the tooth sound, the long sound, the hissing sound, the running sound, the lip-cooler sound, or the "quiet brother" of /v/ (Lindamood and Lindamood, 1998).

Moto-Kinesthetic

With latex gloves, the thumb and forefinger are used to move the lower lip upward until it comes in contact with the upper teeth. Once this position is reached, the client is instructed to blow air (Young and Hawk, 1955).

Sound Approximation

1. Shape /f/ from /p/. Instruct the client to bring the lips together for /p/, then to open them slightly and blow air. Then tell him to bring the lower lip in while he is blowing air. Initially, you may need to maintain correct the articulatory posture with your index finger or a tongue depressor.

2. Shape /f/ from /h/. Have the client prolong /h/ and slowly bring the lips together.

3. Shape /f/ from a whispered /ɑ/. Instruct him to place the lower lip up against the upper teeth as he is saying a whispered (turning off the voice box) /ɑ/.

4. Shape /f/ from /v/. Instruct the client to place one hand on his throat, prolong /v/, and turn off the voicing.

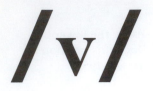

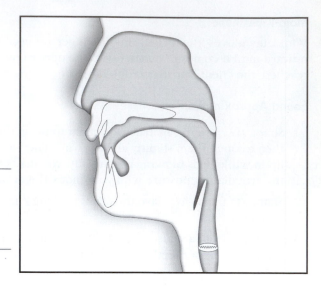

PMV Features:

Labiodental/fricative/
voiced

Production:

As the voiced cognate of /f/, /v/ is produced simi-
larly. The lower edges of the upper teeth are brought into contact with the
lower lip to create a constriction in the oral cavity. The mandible tends to close
so to aid the lower lip in its constricting gesture. The airstream is then directed
through this constriction to produce friction; /v/ is also produced with less
tension than /f/.

Common Errors:

1. Apical-dental: ð/v

2. Bilabial/stop: b/v

3. Bilabial/stop/voiced: p/v

4. Devoicing: f/v

5. Imprecise or improper labiodental contact

6. Voiced bilabial fricative substitution: ß/v

7. Omission

Common Contextual Variants:

Unrounded /v/: village, veal, velvet, involve
Rounded /vʷ/: vote, vocation, avoid, vault, deja vu

Eliciting Techniques:

Phonetic Placement

Demonstrate the feature characteristics of /v/:

- Lower edges of upper teeth lightly contacting the lower lip
- A voiced air stream passing through the small teeth-lip opening
- Velum closed
- Vocal folds vibrating

1. Instruct the client to place his upper teeth on his lower lip and blow air over his lip. Remind him to turn on his voice box.

2. Tell the client to smile slightly and then bite down lightly on his lower lip with his the upper teeth. Hold a strip of lightweight paper in front of his mouth and tell him to blow air lightly while his vocal folds are on. Use a tongue depressor to get the proper shape of the lips and the appropriate opening for the air to pass through.

3. Show the client the exact articulatory position in a mirror. Tell him not to bite on his lip, but to open them slightly and then lightly blow air. Press gently on the client's larynx to signal voicing (turning on the voice box). Instruct the client to lick his lower lip and then to repeat the /v/ production, drawing attention to the air as it cools the lower lip. Label /v/ the Lip Cooler to associate the cooling off of the lip with the sound production (Lindamood and Lindamood, 1998).

4. Instruct the client to his mouth so that the lower lip barely touches his upper teeth. Next, hold his finger crosswise between the lips and blow air. Have the client hold one hand on his throat to feel voicing. Tell him that he can feel the vibration for /v/ on the throat as well as his finger.

5. Practice different labiodental positions. Ask the client to position his upper teeth far down over the lower lip. Have him blow air and gradually move the cutting edges of his upper teeth into the appropriate /v/ placement. Signal voicing by touching the client's throat lightly.

6. Instruct the client to pucker and blow air while he slowly changes the shape of the lips into a smile.

7. Place a small piece of hypo-allergenic tape on the lower lip to develop an awareness of the use of the lower lip.

8. Tell the client to make a "jack-o-lantern" face (Flowers, 1980) while smiling and touching the upper teeth to the lower lips. Position a lightweight strip of paper in front of the client's mouth, then instruct the client to blow out to move it to draw attention to the direction and force of the airflow. Signal turning on the voice box by touching the laryngeal area.

9. As a touch cue, lay the client's finger below his bottom lip.

10. Tell the client to use the jet airplane sound, the housefly sound, the vacuum sweeper sound, the biting lip sound, the tooth sound, the long sound, the hissing sound, the running sound, the lip-cooler sound, or the "noisy brother" of /f/ (Lindamood and Lindamood, 1998).

Moto-Kinesthetic

With latex gloves, the thumb and forefinger are used to move the client's lower lip upward until it comes in contact with the upper teeth. Once this position is reached, instruct the client to blow air. This stimulation is similar to that for /f/ but with firmer contact from the thumb and forefinger. Also, suggest voicing by placing the client's hand on his throat.

Sound Approximation

1. Shape /v/ from /b/. Instruct the client to bring his lips together for /b/. Show him how to vibrate a /b/ at the lips. Then have the client vibrate a /b/ and in so doing retract the lower lip.Initially, you may need to maintain correct articulatory posture with your index finger or a tongue depressor.

2. Shape /v/ from /ɑ/. Instruct the client to place his lower lip against the upper teeth as he is saying /ɑ/.

3. Shape /v/ from /f/. Tell the client to put one hand on his throat, prolong /f/, and turn the vocal folds on while saying /f/.

/θ/

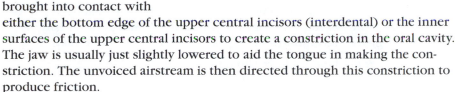

PMV Features:

Lingua (apical) dental/
fricative/voiceless

Production:

The tip of the tongue is
brought into contact with
either the bottom edge of the upper central incisors (interdental) or the inner
surfaces of the upper central incisors to create a constriction in the oral cavity.
The jaw is usually just slightly lowered to aid the tongue in making the constriction. The unvoiced airstream is then directed through this constriction to
produce friction.

Common Errors:

1. Labiodental: f/θ
2. Laminal/alveolar: s/θ
3. Glottal: h/θ
4. Apical-alveolar: t/θ
5. Apical-alveolar/stop/voicing: d/θ
6. Voicing: ð/θ
7. Cosmetic error: acoustically correct but excessive tongue protrusion
8. Omission

Common Contextual Variants:

Unrounded /θ/: thin, think
Rounded /θʷ/: thought, enthusiastic

Dialectal Variations:

f/θ: [fɪn] for thin, [tuf] for tooth
t/θ: [tɪn] for thin, [wɪt] for with

Eliciting Techniques:

Phonetic Placement

Demonstrate the feature characteristics of /θ/:

- Tip of tongue between the upper and lower front teeth, lightly contacting them
- The body of the tongue is relatively flat
- Air forced through the space between the tongue and teeth
- Vocal folds are not vibrating
- Velum closed
- Vocal folds silent

1. Instruct the client to open his teeth slightly and let the tip of his tongue show between the upper and lower teeth. Then, tell him to blow air in a continuous flow down the center of the tongue and between his teeth. Use a tongue depressor to adjust for proper placement. Since /θ/ is easily visible in a mirror, illustrating tongue placement is usually quite easy.

2. Tell the client to hold his lower lip down, slowly stick out his tongue, and then blow air lightly over the tongue.

3. To direct the airflow through the oral cavity, use the following techniques:

   a. Place a straw where the tongue tip contacts the upper and lower front teeth, and have the client direct the air into the straw.

   b. Place the client's finger in front of his lips. Then have him repeat the procedure by himself.

   c. Use a tongue depressor to draw attention to the location of the airstream.

   d. Hold a small strip of lightweight paper in front of the client's mouth near the tongue tip, and ask him to blow out so to make the object move.

4. Tell the client to pretend to cool his tongue after tasting something hot.

5. To control excess tongue protrusion, hold a tongue depressor about one-quarter inch in front of the teeth. If the client can feel the tongue depressor while producing /θ/, the tongue is too far forward.

6. Instruct the client to peek his tongue out between his upper and lower teeth and then slowly and gently close his mouth (retracting the tongue) as he blows out the front of his mouth and cools the tongue.

7. Use a mirror to contrast the client's incorrect production with the correct production.

8. Place a tongue depressor or lollipop directly in front of the client's mouth. Tell the client to touch the object and to gently and gradually close his mouth. You may need to manually assist in closing his jaw so the upper and lower front teeth make lingual contact. Direct the client to blow air over the tongue. Repeat until the client achieves proper tongue protrusion.

9. Tell the client to use the touch cue of placing his finger in front of his lips and remind him to extrude his tongue.

10. Remind the client to use the goose sound, the leaking tire sound, the tongue-teeth sound, tongue-tip sound, the hissing sound, the long sound, the lip-cooler sound, or the "quiet brother" of /ð/ (Lindamood and Lindamood, 1998).

Moto-Kinesthetic

Using latex gloves, the clinician places the jaw in the appropriate position for /θ/. The forefinger of one hand is curved over the upper lip near the central incisors. The thumb and forefinger of the other hand are placed on the chin. Then the tongue is brought into the proper position for /θ/ and the sound is attempted. The clinician moves the lower jaw downward into the next vowel position.

Sound Approximation

1. Shape /θ/ from /s/. Instruct the client to prolong /s/ and slowly slide the tip of the tongue over the upper teeth ("hugging" them with the tip) and then between the teeth.

2. Shape /θ/ from /h/. Tell the client to prolong /h/ and slowly stick his tongue out while gradually closing the mouth.

3. Shape /θ/ from /f/. Instruct the client to produce /f/ in a continuous manner and to "split the /f/ in half" with his tongue by sticking his tongue between his teeth.

4. Shape /θ/ from /t/. Ask the client to slowly release the /t/, creating a friction-like sound. Maintain this quality of production while gliding the tongue over the lower incisors and continuing to direct the airflow over the tongue.

5. Tell the client to say /ð/ while turning off his motor or voice box.

/ð/

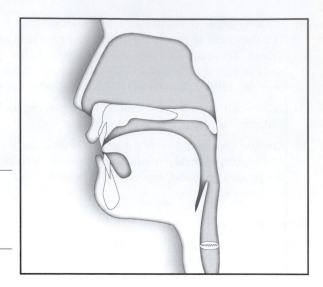

PMV Features:

Lingua (tip) interdental/
fricative/voiced

Production:

As the voiced cognate of
/θ/, /ð/ is produced simi-
larly. The tip of the tongue is brought into contact with either the bottom edge
of the upper and lower central incisors or the inner surfaces of the upper central incisors to create a constriction in the oral cavity. The jaw is usually lowered slightly to aid the tongue in making the constriction. The voiced airstream
is then directed through this constriction to produce friction; /ð/ is also produced with less tension than /θ/.

Common Errors:

1. Labiodental/unvoiced: f/ð
2. Labiodental: v/ð
3. Apical-alveolar: d/ð
4. Laminal-alveolar: z/ð
5. Unvoicing: θ/ð
6. Cosmetic error: acoustically correct but excessive tongue protrusion
7. Excess or insufficient tongue pressure
8. Omission

Common Contextual Variants:

Unrounded /ð/: that, then
Rounded /ðʷ/: although

Dialectal Variations:

v/ð: [vɛn] for then, [beɪv] for bathe
d/ð: [dɛn] for then

Eliciting Techniques:

Phonetic Placement

Demonstrate the feature characteristics of /ð/:

- Tip of tongue between the upper and lower front teeth, lightly contacting them
- The body of the tongue is relatively flat
- Air forced through the space between the tongue and teeth
- Velum closed
- Vocal folds vibrating

1. Instruct the client to open his teeth slightly and let the tip of his tongue show between the upper and lower teeth. Then tell him to blow voiced air in a continuous flow down the center of the tongue and between his teeth. Use a tongue depressor to adjust for proper placement. Since /ð/ is easily visible in a mirror, illustrating tongue placement is usually quite easy.

2. Tell the client to hold the lower lip down, to slowly stick out his tongue, and then to blow air lightly over the tongue. Signal voicing by lightly touching his throat.

3. To direct the airflow through the oral cavity, try the following techniques:

   a. Place a straw where the tongue tip contacts the upper and lower front teeth, and have the client direct the air into the straw.
   b. Place the client's finger in front of his lips. Then have him repeat the procedure by himself.
   c. Use a tongue depressor to draw attention to the location of the airstream.
   d. Hold a small strip of lightweight paper in front of the client's mouth near the tongue tip, and ask him to blow air out to make the object move.

4. Tell the client to pretend to cool his tongue after tasting something hot. Signal voicing by placing his hand on his throat.

5. To control excess tongue protrusion, hold a tongue depressor about one-quarter inch in front of the teeth. If the client can feel the tongue depressor in the production of /ð/, then the tongue is too far forward.

6. Instruct the client to peek his tongue out between his upper and lower teeth and then slowly and gently close his mouth (retracting the tongue) as he blows air out the front of his mouth and cools the tongue. Remind him to turn on his voicing.

7. Use a mirror to contrast the client's incorrect production with the correct production.

8. Place a tongue depressor or lollipop directly in front of the client's mouth. Tell the client to touch the object and to gently and gradually close his mouth. You may need to manually assist in closing his jaw so that the upper and lower front teeth make lingual contact. Direct the client to blow air over the tongue. Repeat until the client achieves proper tongue protrusion. Signal voicing by placing his hand on his throat.

9. Tell the client to use the touch cue of placing his finger in front of his lips, and remind him to extrude his tongue.

10. Remind the client to use the tongue buzzer sound, the motor-on sound, the tongue-teeth sound, the tongue-tip sound, the hissing sound, the long sound, the lip-cooler sound, or the "noisy brother" of /θ/ (Lindamood and Lindamood, 1998).

Moto-Kinesthetic

Using latex gloves, the clinician places the jaw in the appropriate position for /ð/. The forefinger of one hand is curved over the upper lip near the central incisors. The thumb and forefinger of the other hand are placed on the chin. Then the tongue is brought into the proper position for /ð/ (emphasize a firmer contact of the tongue against the teeth than that for /θ/) and the sound is attempted. The clinician moves the lower jaw downward into the next vowel position. Suggest voicing by placing the client's hand on his throat.

Sound Approximation

1. Shape /ð/ from /z/. Instruct the client to prolong /z/, then to slowly slide the tip of the tongue over the upper teeth ("hugging" them with the tip) and then between the teeth.

2. Shape /ð/ from /i/. Tell the client to prolong /i/, then gradually glide the tongue between the teeth to lightly contact his upper teeth with the tongue tip-blade.

3. Shape /ð/ from /v/. Instruct the client to produce /v/ in a continuous manner and to "split the /v/ in half" by sticking his tongue between his teeth.

4. Shape /ð/ from /d/. Instruct the client to vibrate a /d/ (creating a friction-like sound) and then to slowly run the tip of his tongue under the edges of the upper teeth. Remind the client to continue to direct the airstream over the tongue with the voicing (voice motor) on.

5. Tell the client to say /θ/ and turn on his motor or voice box.

/ʃ/

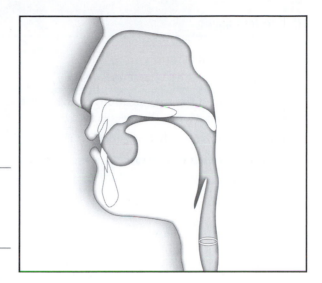

PMV Features:

Palato-alveolar/fricative/
voiceless

Production:

The tongue is raised to
contact the sides with the
upper back teeth, while the blade of the tongue is retracted and almost contacting the front of the palate, creating a broad, shallow groove at the midline
of the tongue. There is a long constriction between the tongue and the roof of
the mouth from just behind the alveolar ridge (where the front of the tongue is
placed) to just in front of the velum (or soft palate). The unvoiced airstream is
directed through this constriction to produce friction. The /ʃ/ sound is usually
rounded, even before front vowels.

Common Errors:

1. Laminal-alveolar: s/ʃ
2. Apical-dental: θ/ʃ
3. Glottal: h/ʃ
4. Voicing: ʒ/ʃ
5. Apical-alveolar/stop: t/ʃ
6. Affricate: tʃ/ʃ
7. Lateral emission: lateral /ʃ/.
8. Omission

Common Contextual Variants:

Although /ʃ/ is most commonly rounded (which serves to lower the frequency
of the noise and help to distinguish it from /s/), individual speakers may have
more or less rounding on the production of /ʃ/, depending on vowels context
(less rounding occurring before unrounded vowels).

Eliciting Techniques:

Phonetic Placement

Demonstrate the feature characteristics of /ʃ/:

- The blade of the tongue almost touches the anterior portion of the palate posterior to the alveolar ridge
- The lips are slightly protruded
- The airstream passes rapidly along a wide medial lingual groove
- Velum closed
- The vocal folds are silent

1. Demonstrate the following procedure step-by-step in a mirror before going through it with the client. You may need to use a tongue depressor to make fine adjustments for place of articulation. Tell the client to:
   a.   Raise the back of the tongue so he can feel his upper teeth.
   b.   Put the tip of the tongue behind his upper teeth, then pull it back a little so he can't feel anything with his tongue tip.
   c.   Pucker his lips a little.
   d.   Blow air slowly over the center of his tongue.

2. Instruct the client to round his lips, flatten his cheeks, and "slush" the air out between his teeth.

3. Rub the upper edges of the tongue with a tongue depressor, sugarless lollipop, or cotton swab. Instruct the client to place the edges of the tongue against the upper teeth and blow air across the blade of his tongue.

4. Instruct the client to fit his tongue around the bowl of a small spoon inserted in his mouth. Have him gradually close his teeth around the handle. This should help him feel the channel necessary for /ʃ/. Tell him to say /ʃ/ with the spoon in his mouth.

5. To develop a central airstream, use any of the following /s/ techniques:
   a.   Forcing air onto a target.
   b.   Holding your fingertip in front of the client's mouth or using his own fingers.
   c.   Directing air through a straw.
   d.   Directing air toward a piece of string or lightweight paper, feather, or pinwheel held in front of the client's mouth.
   e.   Touching the upper molar area with your fingertip on the outside of his cheek to suggest keeping the back of the tongue up.

6. As the client: "What does a person say when they want you to be quiet?" This alone may elicit an approximation of the target sound. Then shape the sound as needed. Add the prompt of holding your index finger straight up and touching your lips as if to make the hushing sound.

7. As a touch cue, lay the client's finger in front of his lips.

8. Remind the client to use the hush sound, the quiet sound, the baby-is-sleeping sound, the seashell sound, the running sound, the flowing sound, the long sound, the back-of-the-hill sound, the fat-air sound, and the "quiet brother" of /ʒ/ (Lindamood and Lindamood, 1998).

Moto-Kinesthetic

Using latex gloves, the clinician places the thumb and forefinger on the corners of the client's upper lip pressing against the upper jaw. The upper lips are then moved toward the center to allow them to protrude slightly.

Sound Approximation

1. Shape /ʃ/ from /n/. Instruct the client to raise the tongue to the position for /n/, to pull the tongue back slightly, to bite down gradually, to pucker a little, and then to blow air.

2. Shape /ʃ/ from /s/.
   a. Have the client prolong /s/, then pull his tongue back slightly and pucker his lips.
   b. Do the same, but guide the movement with a tongue depressor.
   c. Do the same, but with a cotton swab stick inserted between the teeth.

3. Shape /ʃ/ from /θ/-/s/. Have the client prolong /θ/ and slowly bring the tongue inward and upward over the upper teeth, through the position for /s/ and into that for /ʃ/. Have him pucker his lips just before saying /ʃ/.

4. Shape /ʃ/ from /i/-/ɚ/. Instruct the client to prolong /i/, then proceed to /ɚ/ slowly (resulting in something like the word *ear*). Then tell the client to pucker while attempting to say /ʃ/ and turning off the voicing.

5. Shape /ʃ/ from a whispered /ɚ/. Instruct the client to whisper a prolonged /ɚ/ while he brings his teeth together.

6. Shape /ʃ/ from /t-d-n/. Demonstrate a sequence: /t-d-n-/(pucker)-/ʃ/. Allow the client to imitate you. Remind the client to turn off the voicing.

7. Shape /ʃ/ from /t/. Ask the client to prolong the /d/ with lip protrusion. Instruct the client to maintain the protrusion while sliding the tongue backward.

8. Shape /ʃ/ from a whispered /ʒ/. Have the client prolong a whispered /ʒ/ and slowly close his teeth.

9. Shape /ʃ/ from /h/. Have the client prolong /h/, raise his tongue slowly, and pucker his lips.

10. Shape /ʃ/ from /tʃ/.

    a.   Blend a series of rapidly produced /tʃ/ sounds into a /ʃ/.

    b.   Have the client say a /tʃ/ sound slowly, making sure that lip protrusion is occurring during the /ʃ/ production.

11. Shape /ʃ/ from /ʒ/. Instruct the client to place one hand on his throat and to prolong the /ʒ/ sound. Then ask him to stop voicing the sound. Practice voicing and unvoicing.

12. Shape /ʃ/ from /ɑ/ or /i/. Direct the client to say either of the vowels and then to "whisper" the vowel (or turn off the voicing). Next, ask the client to pucker the lips slightly and raise the jaw slightly. Finally, tell him to breathe out while raising the tongue.

/ʒ/

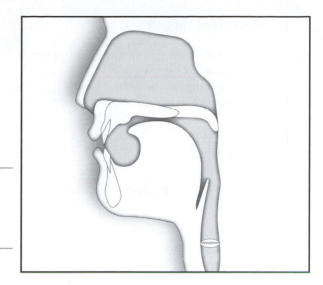

PMV Features:

Palato-alveolar/
fricative/voiced

Production:

As the voiced cognate of
/ʃ/, /ʒ/ is produced simi-
larly. The tongue is raised to contact the sides of the tongue with the upper back
teeth, while the blade of the tongue almost contacts the front of the palate, creating a broad shallow groove at the midline of the tongue. There is a long constriction between the tongue and the roof of the mouth from just behind the alveolar
ridge (where the front of the tongue is placed) to just in front of the velum (or
soft palate). The voiced airstream is directed through this constriction created
by the tongue to produce friction. The /ʒ/ sound is usually rounded, even before
front vowels; /ʒ/ is also produced with less tension than /ʃ/.

Common Errors:

1. Blade-alveolar: z/ʒ
2. Tip-dental: ð/ʒ
3. Tip-dental/unvoiced: θ/ʒ
4. Tip-alveolar/stop: d/ʒ
5. Affricate: dʒ/ʒ
6. Back-velar/stop: g/ʒ
7. Front-palatal/glide: j/ʒ
8. Glottal: h/ʒ
9. Devoicing: ʃ/ʒ
10. Lateral emission: lateral /ʒ/
11. No aperture
12. Omission

Common Contextual Variants:

Although /ʒ/ is most commonly rounded (which serves to lower the frequency of the noise and help to distinguish it from /z/), individual speakers may have more or less rounding on the production of /ʒ/, depending on vowels context (with less rounding before unrounded vowels).

Eliciting Techniques

Phonetic Placement

Demonstrate the feature characteristics of /ʒ/:

- The lips are slightly protruded
- The blade of the tongue almost touches the anterior portion of the palate posterior to the alveolar ridge
- The voiced airstream passes rapidly along a wide medial lingual groove
- Velum closed
- The vocal folds are vibrating

1. Demonstrate the following procedure step-by-step in a mirror first, and then go through it with the client. You may need to use a tongue depressor to make fine adjustments for place of articulation. Tell the client to:
   a. Raise the back of the tongue so he can feel his upper teeth.
   b. Put the tip of the tongue behind his upper teeth, then pull it back a little so he can't feel anything with his tongue tip.
   c. Pucker his lips a little.
   d. Blow voiced air slowly over the center of his tongue.

2. Instruct the client to round his lips, flatten his cheeks, and "slush" the air out between his teeth.

3. Rub the upper edges of the tongue with a tongue depressor, sugarless lollipop, or cotton swab. Instruct the client to place the edges of the tongue against the upper teeth and blow air across the blade of his tongue. Place the client's hand on his throat to feel the vocal fold vibration.

4. Instruct the client to fit his tongue around the bowl of a small spoon inserted in his mouth. Have him gradually close his teeth around the spoon handle. This should help him feel the channel necessary for /ʒ/. Tell him to say /ʒ/ with the spoon in his mouth.

5. To develop a central airstream, use any of the following /s/ techniques:

    a. Forcing air onto a target.

    b. Holding your fingertip in front of the client's mouth or using his own fingers.

    c. Directing air through a straw.

    d. Directing air toward a piece of string or lightweight paper, feather, or pinwheel held in front of the client's mouth.

    e. Touching the upper molar area with your fingertip on the outside of his cheek to suggest keeping the back of the tongue up.

6. As the touch cue, lay the client's finger in front of his lips.

7. Remind the client to use the motor sound, the buzzing saw sound, the running sound, the flowing sound, the long sounds, the back-of-the-hill sound, the fat-air sound, and the "quiet brother" of /ʒ/ (Lindamood and Lindamood, 1998).

Moto-Kinesthetic

Using latex gloves, the clinician places the thumb and forefinger on the corners of the client's upper lip pressing against the upper jaw. The upper lips are then moved toward the center to allow them to protrude slightly. Place the client's hand on his throat to feel vocal cord vibration.

Sound Approximation

1. Shape /ʒ/ from /n/. Instruct the client to raise the tongue to the position for /n/, to pull the tongue back slightly, to bite down gradually, to pucker a little, and to blow air.

2. Shape /ʒ/ from /z/.

    a. Have the client prolong /z/, then pull his tongue back slightly and pucker his lips.

    b. Do the same, but guide the movement with a tongue depressor.

    c. Do the same, but with a cotton swab stick inserted between the teeth.

3. Shape /ʒ/ from /ð/-/z/. Have the client prolong /ð/ and slowly bring the tongue inward and upward over the upper teeth, through the position for /z/ and into that for /ʒ/. Have him pucker his lips just before saying /ʒ/.

4. Shape /ʒ/ from /i/-/ɝ/. Instruct the client to prolong /i/, then proceed to /ɝ/ slowly (resulting in something like the word *ear*), then pucker while attempting to say /ʒ/.

5. Shape /ʒ/ from a whispered /ɝ/. Instruct the client to whisper a prolonged /ɝ/ while he brings his teeth together.

6. Shape /ʒ/ from /t-d-n/. Demonstrate a sequence: /t-d-n/(pucker)-/ʒ/. Allow the client to imitate you.

7. Shape /ʒ/ from /d/. Ask the client to prolong the /d/ with lip protrusion. Instruct the client to maintain the protrusion while sliding the tongue backward.

8. Shape /ʒ/ from /ɚ/. Have the client prolong /ɚ/ and slowly close his teeth.

9. Shape /ʒ/ from /hɑ/. Have the client prolong /hɑ/, raise his tongue slowly, and pucker his lips.

10. Shape /ʒ/ from /dʒ/.

    a.   Blend a series of rapidly produced /dʒ/ sounds into a /ʒ/.

    b.   Have the client say a /dʒ/ sound slowly, making sure that lip protrusion is occurring while prolonging its /ʒ/ component.

11. Shape /ʒ/ from /ʃ/. Instruct the client to place one hand on his throat and prolong the /ʃ/ sound. Then ask him to voice the sound. Practice voicing and unvoicing.

12. Shape /ʒ/ from /ɑ/ or /i/. Direct the client to say either of the vowels. Next, ask the client to pucker the lips slightly while raising the jaw slightly. Finally, tell him to breathe out while raising the tongue.

/h/

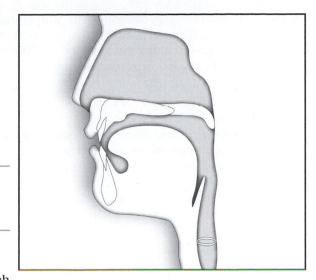

PMV Features:

Glottal/fricative/voiceless

Production:

The vocal folds are posi-
tioned so that they do not
vibrate but are close enough
to produce friction when the airstream passes through the glottis. No particular
articulatory positions are required to produce /h/, although the articulators are
in the position necessary to produce the vowel which follows /h/.

Common Errors:

1. Excessive or insufficient breath pressure
2. Omission

Common Contextual Variants:

Breathy voiced /ɦ/ in intervocal positions: ahoy, ahead, Ahab

Eliciting Techniques:

Phonetic Placement

Demonstrate the features characteristics of /h/:

- Lips assume the position of the sound that will follow
- Tongue is in a neutral position
- Velum closed
- Vocal folds are slightly adducted
- Vocal folds are not vibrating

1. Air is directed through the oral cavity with enough force to create audible friction. The /h/ sound is rarely misarticulated. When it is, the primary difficulty seems to be either too much or too little breath pressure. To overcome this, try the following techniques:

    a. Breathing exercises.

    b. Overemphasis of production at first and then gradual reduction of the amount of air expelled.

    c. Practice directing the air stream onto the client's cupped palm or back of the hand, a pinwheel, a strip of lightweight paper, or a feather. Remind the client to keep the mouth open slightly and tongue relaxed. Have the client continue to repeat the inhalation and exhalation until an acceptable force of air is attained.

    d. Practice saying vowel combinations with varying force (e.g., /a-ha/, /o-ho/, etc.).

2. Point to the larynx while making the /h/ sound.

3. To create the concept of flowing sound, run your hand slowly down your arm while saying a sustained /h/ sound. You can encourage the client to take his hand and imitate the same movement on his own arm.

4. Tell the client to open his mouth and maintain that open posture while blowing the air out of the mouth by pushing the air out with the force chest and abdomen muscles.

5. Contrast the production of "ah" and "ha." It may be helpful to have the client place his hand on his abdomen while producing the two sounds to identify the push of muscles required for production the "ha" which is not needed for the "ah."

6. Remind the client to use the panting dog sound, Santa's "ho-ho-ho" sound, the long sound, the hissing sound, the throat sound, the cousin of the "w" and "wh" sounds, or the wind sound (Lindamood and Lindamood, 1998).

Sound Approximation

1. Shape the /h/ from a forceful exhalation of air. Model the inhalation of air and the forceful exhalation of air. Focus the client on the exhalation of air. Continue to provide guidance until the force of air (audible friction) is within normal limits for /h/.

2. Shape the /h/ from a silent "ah." Tell the client to make a silent "ah." Then have the client maintain an open mouth posture and force some air out of the mouth, resulting in the /h/ sound.

/tʃ/

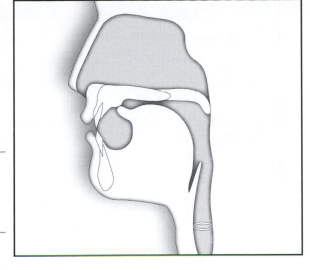

PMV Features:

Palato-alveolar/affricate/
voiceless

Production:

The tip and blade of the
tongue are raised to contact
the post-alveolar ridge, while the sides of the tongue come in contact with the
upper molars to permit a complete stoppage of the airstream. The midline of the
tongue is then suddenly lowered to form a broad shallow constriction as in the /ʃ/
sound. The unvoiced intra-oral breath pressure is released and directed through a
broad point of constriction, producing an explosive friction-like sound.

Common Errors:

1. Tip-dental/fricative: θ/tʃ
2. Blade-alveolar/fricative: s/tʃ
3. Fricative: ʃ/tʃ
4. Tip-alveolar/stop: t/tʃ
5. Back-velar/stop: k/tʃ
6. Voicing: dʒ/tʃ
7. Lateral emission: lateral /tʃ/
8. Omission

Common Contextual Variants:

As with /ʃ/, there may be individual differences in how rounded the /ʃ/ part of
/tʃ/ becomes as a function of vowel context (less rounding before unrounded
vowels).

Eliciting Techniques:

Phonetic Placement

Demonstrate the feature characteristics of /tʃ/:

- The tip of the tongue is raised to the post-alveolar ridge, behind the upper central incisors
- The air pressure is exploded out the mouth through a small opening like that for /ʃ/
- Velum closed
- The vocal folds are silent

1. Using a strip of lightweight paper or a pinwheel, illustrate the plosive release of /tʃ/ on the client's hand. Make sure the client understands that the exploded air is released out the center of the mouth. Place a straw at the center of the client's teeth or hold the client's finger in front of your mouth and then his. This is especially important when the client emits the airstream laterally.

2. Instruct the client to touch his tongue on the "bump" located behind the upper central incisors. You may need to touch the area with a tongue depressor. Next, have him pucker his lips as he lowers the tongue tip and forces air out of the mouth, resulting in /tʃ/. Be sure the tongue assumes a posterior gesture to avoid /ts/. Note that this target sound is produced on a single pulse of air.

3. Illustrations of the tongue positions for /t/ and /ʃ/ are helpful. It is also useful to completely explain how /tʃ/ is composed of /t/ and /ʃ/. Remind the younger child to make the /t/ and /ʃ/ "hold hands," "walk together," or "be friends."

4. Contrast the ease of the airstream for /ʃ/ and the push of the airstream for /tʃ/.

5. Remind the client to use the engine chugging sound, the choo-choo train sound, the sneezing sound, the fat, pushed-air sound, or the "quiet brother" of /dʒ/ (Lindamood and Lindamood, 1998).

Moto-Kinesthetic

Using latex gloves, the clinician places the mouth in the same position as for /ʃ/. The clinician places her thumb and forefinger on the corners of the client's upper lip pressing against the upper jaw. The thumb and forefinger of the other hand are placed just under the lower lip. The lips are held open but the teeth are closed. The clinician then firmly makes the upper lips protrude slightly and quickly brings the lower jaw down with the other hand while removing the hand touching the upper lip (Young and Hawk, 1955).

Sound Approximation

1. Shape /tʃ/ from /t/ and /ʃ/.

   a. Instruct the client to place the teeth and tongue for /t/ and then say the /ʃ/ sound at the same time.

   b. Have the client raise his tongue to the position for /t/. Push the tip back slightly with a tongue depressor to illustrate how to release the pressure.

   c. Tell the client to practice saying /t/-/ʃ/ slowly at first, then rapidly until they blend and become one sound.

2. Instruct the client to practice the exercise /p-t-tʃ/ several times.

3. Instruct the client to practice the exercise /t-ʃ-tʃ/.

4. Shape /tʃ/ from /θ, s, ʃ/.

   a. Instruct the client to prolong /θ/ and retract his tongue to /s/, then /ʃ/. When he says the /ʃ/ sound, tell him to hold that position, inhale more air, and say /tʃ/.

   b. Ask him to attempt the same on one breath.

5. Have the client practice the combination /ʃ-t-ʃ/, slowly at first, then faster.

6. Have the client prolong /ʃ/ and interrupt its flow by elevating the tongue to the position for /t/ and then returning to /ʃ/. This is essentially a slow trilling of /t/ during the continuous production of /ʃ/.

7. Instruct the client to produce a hard /ʃ/.

8. Have the client practice the exercise /s-ʃ-tʃ/.

9. Shape /tʃ/ from /dʒ/. Place the client's hand on his throat. Tell him to practice devoicing /dʒ/, first by prolonging /dʒ/, then by attempting a whispered /dʒ/.

10. Tell the client to imitate the sound of a train, slowly then with increasing speed.

11. Tell the client to imitate the sound of a sneeze: *achoo.*

12. Have the client combine words ending in /t/ and beginning with /j/, e.g., *get you* into *getchu*, *bet you* into *betchu*, *don't you* into *don'tchu*.

13. Shape /t/ from /i/. Instruct the client to close his teeth and prolong /i/, then to raise his tongue up for /t/, and explode air.

14. Have the client make a long /n/ and add /ʃ/. Repeat the combination louder, stronger, faster until the sounds blend and become one sound.

/dʒ/

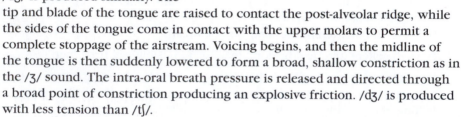

PMV Features:

Palato-alveolar/affricate/voiced

Production:

As the voiced cognate of /tʃ/, /dʒ/ is produced similarly. The tip and blade of the tongue are raised to contact the post-alveolar ridge, while the sides of the tongue come in contact with the upper molars to permit a complete stoppage of the airstream. Voicing begins, and then the midline of the tongue is then suddenly lowered to form a broad, shallow constriction as in the /ʒ/ sound. The intra-oral breath pressure is released and directed through a broad point of constriction producing an explosive friction. /dʒ/ is produced with less tension than /tʃ/.

Common Errors:

1. Tip-dental/fricative: ð/dʒ
2. Tip-dental/fricative/unvoiced: θ/dʒ
3. Fricative: ʒ/dʒ
4. Tip-alveolar/stop: d/dʒ
5. Back-velar/stop: g/dʒ
6. Back-velar/stop/unvoiced: k/dʒ
7. Devoicing: tʃ/dʒ
8. Lateral emission: lateral /dʒ/
9. Omission

Common Contextual Variants:

As with /ʒ/, there may be individual differences in how rounded the /ʒ/ part of /dʒ/ becomes as a function of vowel context (less rounding before unrounded vowels).

Eliciting Techniques:

Phonetic Placement
Demonstrate the feature characteristics of /dʒ/:

- The tip of the tongue is raised to the post-alveolar ridge behind the upper central incisors
- Voiced air pressure explodes out the mouth through a small opening like that for /ʒ/
- The velum is closed
- The vocal folds are vibrating
- The tip of the tongue is raised to the post-alveolar ridge, behind the upper central incisors. The air pressure is exploded out the mouth through a small opening like that for /ʃ/

1. Using a piece of string, lightweight paper, or a feather, illustrate the plosive release of /dʒ/ on the client's hand. Make sure the client understands that the exploded air is released out the center of the mouth. Use a straw at the center of the client's teeth, or hold the client's finger in front of your mouth and then his to show correct placement of the airstream.

2. Instruct the client to touch his tongue on the "bump" located behind the upper central incisors. You may need to touch the area with a tongue depressor. Next, have him pucker his lips as he lowers the tongue tip and forces air out of the mouth, resulting in /dʒ/. Be sure the tongue assumes a posterior gesture to avoid /dz/. Note that this target sound is produced on a single pulse of air.

3. Illustrations of the tongue positions for /d/ and /ʒ/ are helpful. It is good to completely explain how /dʒ/ is composed of /d/ and /ʒ/.

4. Contrast the ease of airflow for /ʒ/ and the push of air for /dʒ/.

5. Give careful instructions regarding voicing. Have the client feel your throat in the production, and place his finger crosswise on your lips to feel a voiced airstream.

6. Remind the client to use the motor-boat sound, the jumping sound, the fat, pushed-air sound, or the "noisy brother" of /ʃ/ (Lindamood and Lindamood, 1998).

Moto-Kinesthetic
Using latex gloves, the clinician positions the client's mouth for /tʃ/. The thumb and forefinger are placed on the corners of the upper lip pressing against the upper jaw. The thumb and forefinger of the other hand are placed just under the lower lip. The lips are held open but the teeth are closed. The clinician then firmly makes the upper lip protrude slightly and slowly brings the lower jaw down

with the other hand while removing the hand touching the upper lip (Young and Hawk, 1955). Place the client's hand on his throat as a reminder for voicing.

Sound Approximation

1. Shape /dʒ/ from /d/ and /ʒ/.

   a. Instruct the client to place the teeth and tongue in the position for /d/ while saying the /ʒ/ sound.

   b. Have the client place the tongue up in the position for /d/. Push the tip back slightly with a tongue depressor to illustrate how to release the pressure.

   c. Tell the client to practice saying /d/-/ʒ/ slowly at first, then rapidly, until they blend and become one sound. Remind the young child to make /d/ and /ʒ/ "hold hands," "be friends," or "walk together."

2. Instruct the client to practice the exercise /b-d-dʒ/.

3. Instruct the client to practice the exercise /d-ʒ-dʒ/.

4. Shape /dʒ/ from /ð, z, ʒ/.

   a. Instruct the client to prolong /ð/ and retract his tongue to /z/, then to /ʒ/. When he says the /ʒ/ sound, tell him to hold that position, inhale more air, and say /dʒ/.

   b. Ask him to attempt the same on one breath.

5. Have the client practice the combination /ʒ-d-ʒ/, slowly at first, then faster.

6. Have the client prolong /ʒ/ and interrupt its flow by elevating the tongue to the position for /d/ and then returning to /ʒ/. This is essentially a slow trilling of /ʒ/ during the continuous production of /ʒ/.

7. Instruct the client to produce a hard /ʒ/.

8. Have the client practice the exercise /z-ʒ-dʒ/.

9. Shape /dʒ/ from /tʃ/. Place the client's hand on his throat and tell him to practice voicing /tʃ/.

10. Place the client's hand on his throat and tell him to imitate the sound of a train. Tell him to voice (i.e., "turn on your motor") those attempts.

11. Have the client combine words ending in /d/ and beginning with /j/, e.g., *had you* into *hadjew*, *need you* into *needjew*.

12. Shape /dʒ/ from /i/. Instruct the client to close his teeth and prolong /i/, then to raise his tongue up for /d/ and explode air.

13. Have the client make a long /n/ and add /ʒ/. Repeat the combination louder, stronger, and faster, until the sounds blend and become one sound.

/m/

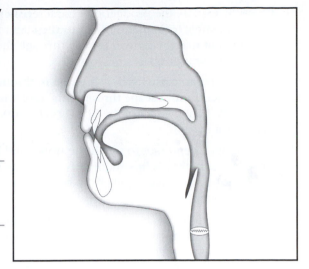

PMV Features:

Bilabial/nasal/voiced

Production:

The lips are pressed together to permit a complete stoppage of the airstream in the oral cavity. The velum is lowered to permit the voiced airstream to escape through the nasal cavity.

Common Errors:

1. Stop (denalization): b/m
2. Stop/unvoiced: p/m
3. Excessive nasality (nasal emission)
4. Omission

Common Contextual Variants:

Unrounded /m/: me, mine, mate, mess
Rounded /mʷ/ (degree of rounding may vary individually): moon, moan, mow
Labio-dental /ɱ/ (in rapid, informal pronunciations): emphatic, emphasis

Eliciting Techniques:

Phonetic Placement

Demonstrate the feature characteristics of /m/:

- Bilabial seal (little tension)
- Nasal emission of air (velum open)
- Vocal cords vibrating

1. Carefully explain the production characteristics using diagrams or illustrations if possible (e.g., pointing out to the client the lip-to-lip posturing, and pointing out that the air will escape through the nose while making the humming sound /m/).

2. Tell the client to close his lips, breathe in through the nose, hold the air, and then let the air escape through his nose while make the /m/ sound. To emphasize light contact of the lips (lip closure), have the client make light kissing sounds.

3. Use a tongue depressor to touch the upper and lower lips. Then instruct the client to close his lips and lightly touch the spot while breathing in through the nose. Ask the client to breath out through the nose to make the /m/ sound.

4. Instruct the client to close his lips and attempt to say /mmmm/. Hold one finger crosswise under his nose to sense nasal emission, or have him lightly pinch his nose to feel vibration. Then, instruct him to lightly press his lips together and then pull his lower jaw down while attempting to say /mɑ/.

5. Ask the client to hum.

6. Elicit an /m/ by asking, "What does one say when a food tasted really good?"----Mmmmmm! (/m/, /m/, /m/, good).

7. Instruct the client to inhale and exhale (breathe) repeatedly. When working with a child, you may find it helps to take turns doing this. Once the breathing pattern is established, instruct the client to hum (add voicing) to the expelled air.

8. To illustrate the amount of pressure on the lips, use your thumb and forefinger to press on his hand. You can also place the back of his forefinger barely between your lips to demonstrate appropriate pressure.

9. As a touch cue, use the client's index finger and thumb to hold his lips together; then ask the client to feel the vibration in his nose.

10. Remind the client to use the humming sound, the cousin of "n" or "ng," or the nose sound (Lindamood and Lindamood, 1998), the taste-good sound, the spinning-top sound, or the voice-box-on or motor-on sound.

Moto-Kinesthetic

Using latex gloves, the clinician places her thumb and forefinger on the client's lower jaw at the center of the lower lip. The lower jaw is brought upward so that the lower lip is lightly touching the upper lip. Touch one finger on the client's nose to signal voicing. Provide an auditory model for the client to produce. When the sound is attempted bring the lower jaw down toward the next vowel sound. *Note:* The upper lip is not touched.

Sound Approximation

1. Shape /m/ from an arrested /ɑ/. Instruct the client to prolong /ɑ/ and arrest it with the bilabial action for /m/ while letting air out through the nose. What results is a sequence similar to /ɑɑɑm-ɑɑɑm-ɑɑɑm/ then /ɑm-ɑm-ɑm-mɑ-mɑ-mɑ-m/. This technique can be used with any vowel.

2. If the client has difficulty sustaining a vowel for technique number 1 above, initiate the vowel with /h/. If he has difficulty timing the sequence, lift his left hand when initiating the production of the vowel and his right on the /m/.

3. Place your forefinger crosswise on the client's lower lip. Instruct him to bring his lips together and hum. Tell him to say /ɑ/ when he feels you push downward on his lip. Make sure he understands to direct the air through the nose.

4. Shape /m/ from /n/. Ask the client to sustain /n/ and then bring his lips together, pulling the tongue and lower jaw down at the same time.

5. Instruct the client to say /bʌ/. Tell the client to continue to make the sound with his lips pressed together while letting the air escape through the nose. You can draw attention to the nasal emission by placing a chilled mirror or piece of lightweight paper under the nostrils.

/ n /

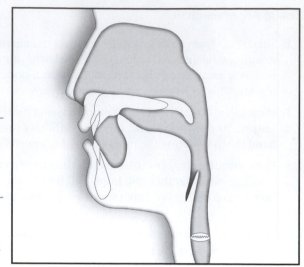

PMV Features:

Lingua (tip) alveolar/
nasal/voiced

Production:

The tip of the tongue is
raised to contact the alveolar ridge behind the central
incisors while the lateral
margins of the tongue con-
tact the lateral upper teeth and gums to permit a complete blockage of the airstream in the oral cavity. The velum is lowered to permit the voiced airstream
to escape through the nasal cavity.

Common Errors:

1. Tip-alveolar/stop (denalization): d/n
2. Bilabial: m/n
3. Tip-dental/fricative: ð/n
4. Back-velar: ŋ/n
5. Tip-alveolar/liquid: l/n
6. Excess tongue pressure
7. Excess nasality (nasal emission)
8. Omission

Common Contextual Variants:

Unrounded /n/: knee, niche, knock, gnat
Rounded /nʷ/ (degree of rounding may vary individually): noon, no, gnaw,
noise
Dental /n̪/: tenth, anthem
Palatal /ɲ/: onion, union

Eliciting Techniques:

Phonetic Placement

Demonstrate the feature characteristics of /n/:

- The tip of the tongue to the alveolar ridge
- Nasal emission of air (velum open)
- Vocal cords vibrating

1. Instruct the client to:
   a. Raise his tongue tip to the ridge just behind the upper teeth. You may assist this action with a tongue depressor.
   b. Lightly touch the end of his nose.
   c. Sustain /n/ directing the voiced air through the nose.
2. To illustrate air passing through the nose, place a small chilled mirror or a piece of lightweight paper under the nostrils. To add the voiced feature, instruct the client to breathe in and out of the nose with the "voice box" or "motor" turned on.
3. Demonstrate nasality that is accompanied with voicing. Ask the client to breathe through his nose, hold it, and say "ah" with the mouth closed, so that the air escapes through the nose.
4. To emphasize the alveolar placement, place some peanut butter (be cautious about food allergies) or flavored food on a cotton swab and touch the "bump" or "hill" behind the upper central incisors. Ask the client to remove the food with the tip of his tongue.
5. /n/ is often elicited in the same manner as /t/ and /d/, except for the nasal emission that is a characteristic of /n/. Please refer to the earlier sections describing the eliciting techniques for /t/ and /d/. Contrast the emission of air through the oral and nasal cavities by using a chilled mirror, feather, or piece of lightweight paper.
6. Use the touch cue of laying the client's forefinger over his cheekbone.
7. Remind the client to use the "no-no" sound, the mosquito sound, the siren sound, the cousin of the /m/ and /ŋ/ sound, or the nose sound (Lindamood and Lindamood, 1998), as well as the bump sound, the hill sound, the voice-box-on sound, or the motor-on sound.

Moto-Kinesthetic

Using latex gloves, hold the client's mouth in the closed position. Place your thumb and forefinger at the corners of the client's lower lip and open the mouth just a little. Then place the forefinger of your other hand on the central bony portion of the nose. Provide an auditory model of /n/. Bring the lower jaw down easily to the position of the next vowel.

Sound Approximation

1. Shape /n/ from an arrested /ɑ/. Instruct the client to prolong /ɑ/ and arrest it with the /n/. First, the client places one hand on his nose and sustains /ɑ/. He then raises his tongue tip to the alveolar ridge to interrupt /ɑ/, then returns to sustaining it. Practice this slowly at first and then faster. What results is a sequence similar to /ɑ . .ɑn. . .ɑ. . ɑn/ then /ɑn-ɑn-ɑn-nɑ-nɑ-nɑ/. This technique can be used with any vowel. The diphthong /aɪ/ is also good to use.

2. Ask the client to practice the sequence /t-d-n/ as in /tɑ-dɑ-nɑ/.

3. Shape /n/ from /m/. Instruct the client to sustain /m/ and slowly raise his tongue to the position for /t/, then open his mouth and pull the tongue back for /ɑ/.

4. Shape /n/ from /ŋ/. Repeat the procedure in number 3 above but use /ŋ/.

5. Shape /n/ from final /l/. Ask the client to sustain /l/, as in the last syllable in *apple*. Instruct the client to make that voiced sound come out the nose and then to pull his tongue down to the position for /ɑ/.

6. Shape the /n/ from /d/. Ask the client to take a deep breath through the nose, hold the air while positioning the tongue in the posture for /d/, and expel the air through the nose while attempting the /n/.

/ŋ/

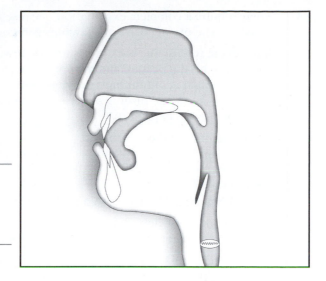

PMV Features:

Lingua (back) velar/
nasal/voiced

Production:

The back of the tongue
is raised to contact the
lowered velum, the second molars, and posterior gum ridges to prevent
the airstream from entering the oral cavity. The velum is lowered to permit
the voiced airstream to escape through the nasal cavity. The vocal folds are
adducted.

Common Errors:

1. Tip-alveolar (denalization): n/ŋ
2. Stop: g/ŋ (denasalization)
3. Excess nasality (nasal emission)
4. Omission

Common Contextual Variants:

The sound /ŋ/ occurs only following a vowel in syllable coda position in
English, and thus one finds little contextual variation as a function of vowel
context. However, as a function of social dialect, some speakers may add a /g/
in the production of a word such as hung (/hʌŋg/).

Eliciting Techniques:

Phonetic Placement

Demonstrate the feature characteristics of /ŋ/:

- Back of the tongue contacts the soft palate
- Air stream emitted through the nose (velum open)
- Vocal folds vibrating

1. /ŋ/ may require a complete explanation because the place of articulation is less visible. The use of charts or drawings is recommended.

2. Ask the client to raise the back of his tongue toward the back of his mouth. Compare it with the posture and movement of /k/ or /g/. Then instruct the client to breathe out through the nose while voicing. For the child, you may want to say "while turning on your voice box." Various tactile strategies can be used to explain /ŋ/:

   a. Holding one hand on the nose.
   b. Putting both hands on the underside of the jaw where it meets the neck.
   c. Swallowing.
   d. Touching the soft palate with a tongue depressor.

3. To illustrate nasal air flow, hold a chilled mirror, feather, lightweight piece of paper, or the client's forefinger crosswise under the client's nose.

4. Instruct the client to hum, say /m/, or say "ah" with the mouth closed. Demonstrate the positioning of the tongue for /ŋ/. Then instruct the client to raise the back of the tongue while resting the tip behind the lower central incisors. Finally, ask the client once again to say /m/, or say "ah" with the mouth closed and without moving the tongue out of position.

5. Ask the client to listen to the difference between /n/ and /ŋ/. Open your mouth while saying each of the sounds, and point out the position of the tip of the tongue when making the /n/ and the position of the back of the tongue for making the /ŋ/.

6. Contrast the oral positions for the production of /m/, /n/, and /ŋ/. Gesture with your index finger at the lips and then along the cheek as you refer to each of the three nasal sounds. Refer to the sounds as the front, middle, and back cousins (Lindamood and Lindamood, 1998).

7. As a touch cue, instruct the client to lay his forefinger on the upper most part of the neck.

8. Remind the client to use the gong sound, the electric-wire sound, the voice-on sound, the nose sound, and the cousin of /n/ and /m/ (Lindamood and Lindamood, 1998).

Moto-Kinesthetic

Using latex gloves, the clinician places the thumb and forefinger on the throat at the base of the tongue. The jaw is lowered. Press gently upward while holding the other hand on the nose. Ask the client to imitate your model of /ŋ/.

Sound Approximation

1. Shape /ŋ/ from /g/ or /k/. Those sounds are good to teach placement. Ask the client to prolong a nasal /ɑ/ and arrest it with /g/. If this does not work, try /k/. Another approach is asking the client to say /g/ or /k/ with the mouth closed, thus directing the nasal emission.

2. Have the client practice the sequence /m/-/n/-/ŋ/.

3. Shape /ŋ/ from /n/:

   a. Instruct the client to place the tip of his tongue behind the lower teeth. You may need to hold the front of the tongue down with a tongue depressor. Ask the client to say /n/. What may result is a palatal /ŋ/.

   b. Ask the client to open his mouth wide. Hold his lower jaw down so that his tongue cannot reach the alveolar ridge. Then ask the client to say /n/.

   c. Tell the client to sustain /n/ and swallow a /g/ sound.

   d. Ask him to sustain /n/ and make a whispered /k/.

   e. Instruct him to sustain /n/ into a whispered, slowly said cough.

4. Tell the client to sustain the /i/ sound, then raise the back of the tongue while forming a seal with the posterior roof of the mouth. Repeat the direction, calling attention to the tongue placement and nasal emission.

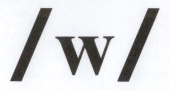

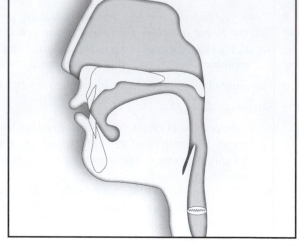

PMV Features:

Labio-velar/glide/voiced

Production:

The back of the tongue is raised to the velum but does not contact the velum, and the lips are rounded. The voiced airstream is directed through the lips, while the articulators (lips and tongue) suddenly shift to assume the position necessary to produce the vowel sound which follows /w/.

Common Errors:

1. Stop: b/w
2. Stop/unvoiced: p/w
3. Labiodental/fricative: v/w
4. Omission

Common Contextual Variants:

Some dialects, notably Appalachian English, contrast between /w/ and /ʍ/ (/hw/) in word pairs like witch (/wɪtʃ/) and which (/ʍɪtʃ/); wear (/wɛɚ/) and where (/ʍɛɚ/); and watt(/wɑt/) and what (/ʍɑt/ or /hwɑt/).

Eliciting Techniques:

Phonetic Placement

Demonstrate the feature characteristics of /w/:

- Bilabial rounding and movement toward the lip position required for the next vowel
- High back tongue posture, moving toward the tongue position for the next vowel

- Voiced airstream emitted through the rounded lips
- Velum opened
- Vocal folds vibrating

1. Show the client the shape of the lips to initiate /w/. Ask the client to round his lips and place them close together. Next, tell the client to raise the very back of the tongue toward the posterior roof of this mouth. Labial and lingual positioning can be indicated by a tongue depressor. Finally, instruct the client to exhale through the oral cavity, resulting in a /wu/.

2. Explain that the tongue placement necessary to begin /w/ approximates that position required for the vowel /u/.

3. Explain that /w/ always begins near /u/ and ends at the vowel that follows. Placement is not static, however. Show the client that his lips take a rounded position at first and then take the shape necessary to utter the next vowel. For example:

   /wi/—lips begin rounded but end unrounded.
   /wu/—lips begin rounded and remain rounded to produce /u/.

4. Place the client's gloved hand on your lips to allow him to feel the difference in lip movement and a gliding movement toward the next vowel.

5. To give the client the sense of the length of this sound, run your hand down the length of your arm, or have him do this to his or your arm.

6. Remind the client to use the "wow" sound, the round lip sound, the front sound, the crying-baby "wah-wah" sound, the wind sound, or the cousin of the "h" and "wh" sounds (Lindamood and Lindamood, 1998).

Moto-Kinesthetic

Using latex gloves, place the thumb and forefinger of one hand on the client's upper lip and the thumb and forefinger of the other hand on the lower lip. Bring the lips together to a rounded position (approximately that for /u/) so that a small opening remains. Instruct the client to say /u/. Then bring the lower jaw into the position required for the next vowel.

Sound Approximation

1. Shape /w/ from /u/. While the client is saying /u/, ask him to close his lips, resulting in the /w/. Another approach is to have the client practice syllables that begin with /u/ and terminate with another vowel:

   a. To contrast the rounding and unrounding, start with /u/ and use unrounded vowels, e.g., /uwi/, /uwe/, uwɑ/.
   b. Then move to /u/ with central vowels, e.g., /uwʌ/, /uwɚ/.
   c. Finally, practice /u/ with rounded vowels, e.g., /uwɚ/, /uwo/, /uwu/.

2. A variation is to ask the client to practice progressively closer sequences of /u/ followed by another unrounded vowel, /u/ . . /ɑ/, /u/ . . . /ɑ/, /u/ . . /ɑ/, /uwɑ/. When the arresting vowel approximates /u/, the clinician can quickly stroke the client's lower lip. Rapid productions of /u/-/ɑ/ typically result in /wɑ, wɑ, wɑ, wɑ/.

3. Shape from /bu/ to /wu/. Have the client say /bu/ and then round his lip, puckering them slightly. Tell the client to attempt to say /bu/, resulting in /wu/.

4. Have the client say the following sequence rapidly /u/ + /ɑ/, resulting in /uwɑ/. Once the /uwɑ/ is established, fade the /u/ by "making the /u/ silent" which will result in /wɑ/.

/j/

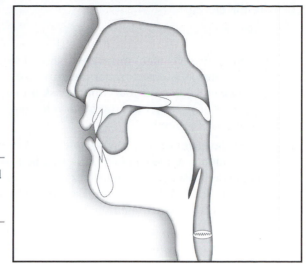

PMV Features:

Lingua-palatal/glide/voiced

Production:

The tip and blade of the tongue are raised toward the palate but do not contact the palate. Then the tongue suddenly shifts to the position necessary to produce the vowel following /j/, while the voiced airstream is directed over the top of the tongue.

Common Errors:

1. Tip-alveolar: l/j
2. Bilabial glide: w/j
3. Omission

Common Contextual Variants:

Unrounded /j/: yet, yak, yacht, yes
Rounded /jʷ/: you, youth, yoke, yawn
Voiceless /j̥/: cue, cute, puke, puce

Eliciting Techniques:

Phonetic Placement:

Demonstrate the feature characteristics of /j/:

- Tongue positioned to start the sound near that required for the high-front vowel /i/
- Voiced airstream passes over the elevated portion of the tongue as it glides to assume the position of the next vowel

- Velum closed
- Vocal folds vibrating

1. Most phonetic placement techniques should focus on showing the client that /j/ begins as a tense form of the vowel /i/. Have the client observe the difference in tension on your mouth. Ask him to also sense the movements of the sides of your lips and the motion of your jaw as you arrest /j/ with the vowel that follows.

2. Instruct the client to relax the tongue flat in the tongue. Have the client open his mouth while you touch the middle portion of the tongue with a tongue depressor, and then instruct the client to raise the touched area slightly (for the child refer to the area as the "magic spot"). Finally, tell the client to breathe out through the mouth, resulting in /j/.

3. Remind the client to use the yes sound, the yo-yo sound, the flowing sound, the middle sound, the voice-is-on sound, or the motor-is-on sound.

Moto-Kinesthetic

Use latex gloves. For clients with normal occlusion, bring the teeth together and then separate them slightly so that the incisors show. Apply pressure with the thumb and forefinger of one hand to the corners of the upper lip. Hold the lower jaw with the thumb and forefinger of the other hand at the corners of the lower lip. Instruct the client to say /i/ as you apply pressure to the upper lip, then move the lower jaw downward.

Sound Approximation

1. Shape /j/ from /i/.

   a. Instruct the client to prolong /i/ and then say /ɑ/ or /u/:

      /i/-/jɑ/ (yah)
      /i/-/ju/ (you)

   b. Instruct the client to place his tongue in the position for /i/, but without actually saying /i/ ("think it" instead of saying it). Then ask him to say /jɑ/ or /ju/.

   c. A variation of the exercise above is to begin /j/ with a whispered /i/.

2. Tell the client to say /ʒ/ rapidly. This often results in /j/. Instruct the client to lower the tongue, and remind him that the movement should be quick and tense.

3. Ask the client to sustain /ð/ while retracting the tongue until the tip of the tongue is positioned even with the back portion of the alveolar ridge. Then have the client lower the lingual tip while breathing out of the oral cavity to produce /j/.

/l/

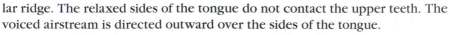

PMV Features:

Lingua (tip) alveolar/
liquid/ voiced

Production:

The tip of the tongue is
raised to contact the alveo-
lar ridge. The relaxed sides of the tongue do not contact the upper teeth. The
voiced airstream is directed outward over the sides of the tongue.

Common Errors:

1. Bilabial: w/l
2. Front-palatal: j/l
3. Central-palatal: r/l
4. Back-velar/stop: g/l
5. Tip-dental/fricative: ð/l
6. Insufficient or excess tongue pressure (voiced lateral fricative)
7. Blade-alveolar placement
8. Omission

Common Contextual Variants:

Unrounded /l/: like, let, leak, lack
Rounded /lʷ/: Lou, look, low
Voiceless /l̥/: please, plus, clue, clap

Eliciting Techniques

Phonetic Placement

Demonstrate the feature characteristics of /l/:

- Tongue tip touching and releasing the alveolar ridge
- Voiced airstream passing over the sides of the tongue
- Velum closed
- Vocal folds vibrating

1. Show the client the correct tongue placement and movement:

   a.   Lightly brush the alveolar ridge with the tip of a tongue depressor, and ask him to put his tongue tip on that spot and then to say /lɑ/. Be sure to monitor the forward positioning of the dorsum of the tongue so that the tip of the tongue is contacting the alveolar ridge.

   b.   Dampen the end of a cotton swab and rub the cotton portion over flavored hard candy; then touch the alveolar ridge with the swab to have him "taste" the correct placement.

   c.   As a variation of (b) above, apply peanut butter or use a lollipop to touch the alveolar ridge; or place a small piece of hard candy on the alveolar ridge ("magic spot"). Be sure not to use a food that may cause an allergic reaction.

   d.   Have the client practice raising and lowering the tongue tip first slowly and then faster to the alveolar ridge. Make sure his mouth is open wide so that you can check placement.

   e.   Instruct the client to feel his tongue with his fingertip as he moves it up and down.

   f.   Guide the tongue movement to and from the alveolar ridge with a tongue depressor.

   g.   Ask the client to feel the bump or hill behind his upper front teeth.

2. Instruct the client to place one hand on your throat as you say /l/ to feel voicing.

3. Tell the client to make a flat tongue and then raise the tip of the flattened tongue to the spot behind the upper front teeth. Remind the client that there is no lip rounding. Avoid using /l/ with rounded vowels (e.g., /u/).

4. To monitor the movement of a flattened versus rolled tongue, have the client assume a wide-open mouth posture while looking into a mirror. Once the client can achieve the flattened tongue posturing, instruct him to raise the tip of the tongue on the alveolar ridge behind the upper front teeth.

5. Place a straw at the corner of the mouth or along the lateral teeth to demonstrate the lateral emission of air. Draw attention to the lateral emission of air by calling attention to the cool air felt on the sides of the tongue as the /l/ is being produced. To emphasize the air-cooling sensation, first

have the client suck on a piece of peppermint candy for a few minutes before doing this exercise.

6. First place a half-inch-wide ribbon across the front of the tongue so that the ends hang down to the client's chin. Then instruct the client to touch the alveolar ridge behind the upper central incisors. Next, instruct the client to say /l/ while you gently pull down the sides of the ribbon allowing the lateral airflow (Bauman-Waengler, 2004).

7. Contrast the lip posturing for /w/ and /l/. For /w/, show (explain) the client that the lips are rounded and protruded; but for the /l/, the lips are separated and somewhat relaxed.

8. As a touch cue, lay the client's fingertip on the middle of his upper lip.

9. Remind the client to use the singing sound (la la), the lullaby sound, the pointy sound, the tongue-tip sound, the flowing sound, the bump sound, the hill sound, or the lifter sound (Lindamood and Lindamood, 1998).

Moto-Kinesthetic

Part 1: Using latex gloves, the clinician sets the client's mouth slightly open. The thumb and forefinger of one hand are placed three-fourths to one inch apart from each other at the center of the upper lip. Pressure is applied there first to stimulate vocalic /l/.

Part 2: The thumb and forefinger of the other hand are placed similarly under the lower lip. After the vocalic /l/ begins, the lower jaw is moved quickly downward toward the next vowel.

Sound Approximation

1. /l/ from /ɑ/.

   a. Instruct the client to prolong /ɑ/ and interrupt its production by raising his tongue tip to the alveolar ridge (e.g., /ɑ . . . lɑ . . . lɑ . . . lɑ/).
   b. Ask him to prolong /ɑ/ and gradually lift the tongue to the alveolar ridge and remove it quickly.
   c. Instruct the client to whisper /ɑ/ while he places his tongue tip on the alveolar ridge. Then tell him to say /ɑ/ very loudly and release his tongue.

2. Shape final /l/ from /i/.

   a. Instruct the client to prolong /i/ and raise the tongue tip to the alveolar ridge while slowly opening the mouth wider. This should produce /i/. This exercise can also be done from /ɑ/, with the mouth in a position less open than normal.
   b. Instruct the client to prolong /i/ and use his tongue to brush the area just behind the teeth with his tongue. For a young child, use the analogy of painting with a paintbrush or licking a lollipop.

3. Have the client practice the sequence /t/-/d/-/n/-/l/.

4. Shape /l/ from /n/. Have the client practice the sequence /nɑ/-/lɑ/, /nɑ/-/lɑ/.

5. Shape /l/ from /t/. Have the client practice the sequence /ti/-/li/, /ti/-/li/. This exercise can also be done from /d/.

6. Shape /l/ from /ŏ/. Instruct the client to say /ŏ/. Then tell the client to lower the jaw and draw the tongue tip backward until it contacts the alveolar ridge behind the upper front teeth. While maintaining contact with the alveolar ridge, the client says /l/.

7. Shape light (front) /l/ from /i/. Direct the client to keep the tongue in the position of /i/ while attempting /ɑ/, which will result in a light /l/.

8. Shape final /l/ from /ʌ/. Instruct the client to raise his tongue to the alveolar ridge and prolong /ʌ/.

9. Shape a dark (back) /l/. Direct the client to keep the tongue in the position of /u/ while attempting /ɑ/, which will result in a dark /ɫ/.

A Final Note: Because /w/ is so frequently substituted for /l/, you may need to inhibit bilabial movement by placing your gloved hands on the client's lips, by using a tongue depressor, or by having the client retract his lips first.

/r/

This section approaches the sound /r/ from two different viewpoints, depending on whether the sound occurs in the prevocalic position (a "consonantal" /r/) or in postvocalic (syllable coda) position, in which it is more like the diphthongal off-glide schwar /ɝ/.

Prevocalic /r/ (/ɹ/)

A prevocalic /r/ occurs either in syllabic initial position (as in *read, read, raw*) or as the last element in a prevocalic consonant cluster (as in *pray, tray, shred, strain*). Most phoneticians describe the prevocalic /r/ as produced as a retroflex glide (in narrow IPA transcription: /ɻ/) or as a bunched tongue /r/ (in narrow IPA transcription: /ɹ/). In practice, these two different productions sound identical (even to a well-trained ear). For this reason, we will use the phonetic symbol /r/[2] to refer to this prevocalic rhotic[3] sound. Because of the complexity of the /r/ sound, an entire chapter this book is completely devoted to describing how it is produced.

---

[2] Technically, the phonetic symbol /r/ in IPA transcription represents a trilled /r/ (as found in Spanish). However, since there is no trilled /r/ in American English, it is usual to use this symbol to refer to both /ɻ/ and /ɹ/.

[3] The term "rhotic" is an acoustic term which refers to a lowered third formant. However, all sounds with this property are "r-colored"; that is, they sound as if they have an /r/ in them. The related term *retroflex* is an articulatory term that means that the tongue tip is curled back when the sound is produced. All retroflex sounds are both rhotic and r-colored. However, not all rhotic or r-colored sounds are retroflexed. For example, the bunched tongue /r/ is rhotic and r-colored, but not retroflexed.

Retroflex /r/ (/ɭ/ or /ɻ/)

Production:

The body of the tongue is raised toward the palate, with the tip raised to approximate the alveolar ridge or prepalatal area. The tip of the tongue is typically slightly curl ed up and bent backward. The edges of the tongue are raised. The voiced airstream is released over the top of the tongue. Lip rounding may be present.

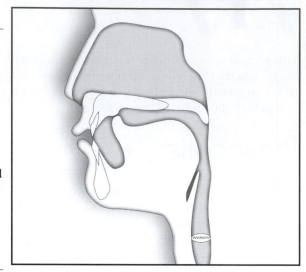

PMV Features:

Apical-prepalatal voiced liquid

Bunched Tongue /r/ (/ɻ/)

Production:

The body of the tongue is raised toward the palate, with the tip of the tongue pointing down toward the lower teeth, and the sides of the tongue touching the upper bicuspids and molars. The voiced airstream is released over the top of the tongue. Lip rounding may be present.

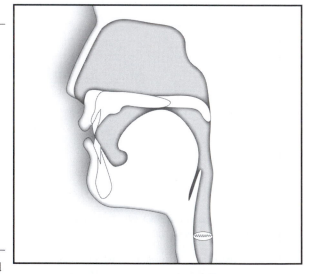

PMV Features:

Dorsal-palatal voiced liquid

Common Errors:

1. Bilabial: w/r
2. Front-palatal: j/r
3. Tip-alveolar: l/r
4. Vowels replace the r-colored central vowels (see the following comments)
5. Omission

Common Contextual Variants:

Voiceless /r̥/: train, pray, crutch, cry

Eliciting Techniques:

Phonetic Placement

Demonstrate the feature characteristics of either the bunched or retroflexed/rhotacized /r/:

- Tongue tip raised and curled upward pointing just behind the alveolar ridge but not touching it, or tip is pointed downward toward the lower teeth
- The corpus of the tongue is raised toward the palate
- Voiced airstream released over the tongue as it glides toward the position of the next vowel
- Velum closed
- Vocal folds vibrating

Clinical Note: The articulation of the /r/ is highly variable, with the production being significantly influenced by its context. Either of the two broad possibilities described above will be referred to in the following suggested techniques. The attending speech-language pathologist should select the techniques most relevant to the client's approximated production and/or stimulability. In addition, some clients generalize the correct production of the vocalic "r" to the correct production of the consonantal /r/, which suggests that the vocalic "r" should be established before introducing the production of the consonantal /r/.

1. Show the client how to raise the tongue (i.e., curl the tongue upward or point the tongue downward in the retroflexed and bunched posture respectively). Use a tongue depressor to guide the movement if necessary. Hold the lips still to focus attention on the tongue movement.
2. Illustrations of tongue placement are helpful for some individuals. Try demonstrating the tongue movement with your hands. Hold one hand horizontally to represent the tongue. With your other hand underneath to

represent the floor of the mouth, demonstrate the tongue movement for /r/ (e.g., bunched posture). As another illustration, have the client cup his hand to mimic the tongue tip raised and slightly curled back (e.g., retroflexed posture).

3. Tell the client to place his tongue tip behind his upper front teeth. Using a tongue depressor, place the lingual tip on the "shelf" made by the depressor and lift it to help the client position the tongue correctly. Next, instruct the client to curl the tongue backward without touching the roof of the mouth until it cannot go back any farther. Finally, tell the client to lower the jaw slightly and attempt /ru/ (e.g., retroflexed posture).

4. To establish the retroflex /r/, Bauman-Waengler (2004) recommends a "sweeping" action using the following steps:

   a. Show the client how to raise the tongue behind the alveolar ridge without making contact with this articulator.
   b. Have the client raise the posterior edges of the tongue to touch the upper molars.
   c. Introduce movement by having the client "sweep" the palatal area. Instruct him to glide the tongue while touching the alveolar area, backward and forward, while "sweeping" the palatal area.
   d. Have the client open his mouth slightly and repeat the sweeping movement without touching the tip of the tongue or palatal area, while keeping the edges of the tongue raised and adding voicing. As the tongue edges are raised and voicing is added, an r-like quality is produced.

5. Direct the client to stick out his tongue. With a tongue depressor, touch the edges of the tongue. Then use the depressor to touch the gum areas alongside the upper molars. Next, tell the client to bring the tongue back into the mouth while raising the tongue, to make the edges of his tongue contact the upper teeth where you just touched (e.g., bunched posture).

6. To inhibit /w/:

   a. Retract the lips slightly. Suggest trying a "small smile," or say "let the lips go to sleep," or "no kissing frogs."
   b. Place the client's forefinger crosswise on his lower lip. Tell him to concentrate on his tongue and to move the whole body of the tongue forward.
   c. Position the mouth in a somewhat open position but not so open that it interferes with the tongue elevation.

7. To inhibit the /j/ (tongue is convex for /j/, Bauman-Waengler, 2004):

   a. Position the mouth in a more open posture.
   b. Roll the tongue to achieve a medial lingual groove.

8. To inhibit the /l/:

   a. Release the tongue tip from the alveolar ridge.

b. Raise the edges for the tongue to prevent lateral airflow.

c. Move the tongue slightly backward.

9. Remind the client to use the growling dog sound (grrr), the tiger sound (grrr), the growling sound, the rac ecar sound (ruh), the middle sound, the flowing sound, or the lifter sound (Lindamood and Lindamood, 1998).

Moto-Kinesthetic

Using latex gloves, the clinician places the thumb and forefinger of one hand on the upper lip about an inch apart. The thumb and forefinger of the other hand are placed similarly on the lower lip. The mouth is open slightly to make the tongue visible. The lips are held firmly to inhibit rounding. When the /r/ is attempted, the lower jaw is moved downward toward the next vowel (Young and Hawk, 1955).

Sound Approximation

1. Shape /r/ from /ɝ/. Practice syllables that begin with /ɝ/ (e.g., /ɝra, ɝri, ɝro/). *Warning:* Beware of the risk of teaching the client to precede all consonant /r/ words with /ɝ/. If you use this exercise, teach the client to whisper /ɝ/ before the consonant /r/.

2. Separate /r/ from intervocalic /ɝr/ contexts that occur in certain words. The intervocalic /ɝr/ contains both the vocalic /ɝ/ and the consonant /r/. Individuals who can say or who have been taught the vowel first but say w/r often produce /r/ correctly in intervocalic contexts. Use these contexts to begin training (Slipakoff, 1967). For example:

   carry ⇒ care re ⇒ care read ⇒ read
   caring ⇒ care ring ⇒ ring

   For children, Garbutt and Anderson (1980) suggest distinguishing between two kinds of "R's," the standing R and the running R. They can be located in words containing the intervocalic /ɝr/ as in *marry*, *carry*, and *carrot*. The standing R "purrs" as in *her*. The running R as in *run* begins with the standing R. It needs the standing R to make it run.

3. Shape /r/ from /ʒ/. Instruct him to prolong /ʒ/ and then stop while holding that tongue position, think a silent /ɝ/ or /ʌ/, and say /rʌ/.

4. Have the client practice the sequence /tʌ-dʌ-lʌ-rʌ/.

5. Shape /r/ from /t/ or /d/. Practice sequences /tʌ rʌ/→ /tɝ/ → /tr/. Instruct the client to pull his tongue back slightly while pointing the tongue tip in the direction of the pre-palatal area; then lift the edges of the tongue to touch the back upper back teeth and say /r/ with emphasis.

6. Shape /r/ from /n/. Practice saying *none* (tongue back) *run*, and practice saying /nʌ-rə/ or /nə/-*run*.

7. Insert a silent /ɝ/ between /t/ and /r/ and /d/ and /r/ blends. Instruct the client to say *train, tree* or *dream, dry,* and insert a silent or whispered /ɝ/ after the initial consonant.

Postvocalic /ɚ/

Common Errors:

The primary error on all variations of vocalic "R" is an absence of /ɚ/ resonance. This usually results because the individual fails to either bulge (bunch) the central portion of the tongue or retroflex it. Frequent errors are

/bud/ for /bɝd/ (bird)
/mudu/ for /mɝdɚ/ (murder)
/fum/ for /faɚm/ (farm)
/hɛu/ for /hɛɚ/ (hair)
/faɪu/ for /faɪɚ/ (fire)

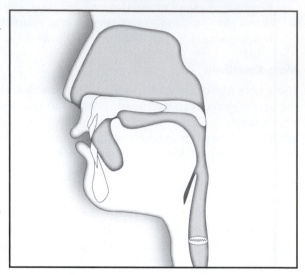

A postvocalic /r/ (for which we will use the schwar symbol, /ɚ/) is much more vowel-like than the prevocalic /r/ and can be produced using either the bunched tongue or retroflex gestures. Note that the postvocalic /ɚ/ acts like the off-glide of a diphthong and is consequently very "vowel-like." Examples of words with postvocalic /ɚ/ include *bear* (/bɛɚ/), *sore* (/sɔɚ/), and *far* (/faɚ/). Normally, the postvocalic /ɚ/ does not constitute a syllable peak by itself, and thus *bear*, *sore*, and *far* are one-syllable words. However, individual variation may make the postvocalic /ɚ/ into a distinct syllable. In that case, the word has two syllables (e.g., the difference between *bear* and *Bayer*).

Common Contextual Variants:

Some individuals (and some dialects) do not produce post-vocalic /r/'s (e.g., many New England dialects). In these cases, /ə/ is produced as the off-glide instead of /ɚ/.

Eliciting Techniques:

1. Shriberg (1975) suggests seven articulatory requisites for /ɚ/:
   a. Be able to move the body of the tongue grossly on command.
   b. Know (by pointing with his finger) where his tongue tip is.
   c. Know (by pointing) where his alveolar ridge is.
   d. Be able to lift his tongue tip to his alveolar ridge.

    e.   Be able to sustain elevation of his tongue tip for several seconds (at least five) without the tongue tip roving around.

    f.   Be able to move tongue body and tip forward and backward without jaw motion.

    g.   Be able to move and tense his tongue independently of phonation jaw movement.

2. Instruct the client to growl like a tiger while you model the /ɝ/, to make a sound like a motor starting up.

3. Have the client lie his back on a floor mat, relax the mouth, and say /ɝ/.

4. Direct the client to lower the tongue tip and the draw the back of the tongue posteriorly, as for producing a silent /g/. Then tell the client to make the edges of the tongue touch the insides of the back teeth. Remind the client to turn on the voice box while producing /ɝ/.

5. Tell the client to open his mouth and make a silent /k/, and then attempt a growling sound /ɝ/.

6. Tell the client to open his mouth and to raise the tongue. Model the tongue tip in the center of the mouth almost touching the hard palate. Use a mirror to improve the demonstration. Then direct the client to close his mouth until his teeth are almost clenched, and then say /ɝ/ (e.g., retroflexed posture).

7. Tell the client that you are going to pull on an imaginary string attached to the back of his head. As you pull the imaginary string up from the back of the client's head, instruct the client to lift the back of a tensed tongue and say /ɝ/. For the younger client, you may want to introduce this task by asking him to pretend he is a puppet (e.g., bunched posture).

8. Show the client the shape of the lips and the height of the tongue in the production of /ɝ/. Have him feel the vibration on in his throat about where you would stimulate /k/. Although many clinicians focus on retracting the tongue tip, we believe you should show the height of the back of the tongue. Demonstrate by placing the tip of your tongue down behind your lower teeth and saying /ɝ/ to show the elevation of the back of the tongue (e.g., bunched posture). Also demonstrate the articulatory posture by showing the retraction of the tongue tip (e.g., retroflexed posture).

9. Use a tongue depressor to help the client attain the /ɝ/ posture. Slowly move the tongue back while the client is attempting to produce /ɝ/. Place the tip of a tongue depressor on the gum ridge behind the lower central incisors and ask the client to hold it there with the underside of the tongue. Move the tongue back with a lever action of the tongue depressor while the client is attempting /ɝ/.

10. Show a curling movement of the tongue with your hands. Hold one hand out palm down to represent the tongue, and place the other hand underneath to represent the floor of the mouth. Move the upper hand to illustrate the backward curling action. You can also hold your hand out palm

up and gradually make your fingers curl upward to show the upward curling action. Have the client try this while attempting to produce /ɚ/. Some clients produce excessive lip rounding. To minimize the lip rounding, place your thumb and forefingers at the corners of the client's lower lip, or lay a tongue depressor crosswise on his lower lip.

11. Tell the client that you are going to pull an imaginary string attached to the back of his head. As you pull the imaginary string up from the back of the client's head, instruct the client to lift the back of a tensed tongue and say /ɚ/. For the younger client, you may want to introduce this task by asking him to pretend he is a puppet (e.g., bunched posture).

12. Tell the client to place his tongue tip on the roof of his mouth and then drop it slightly while saying /ɚ/. *Note*: Be careful when you emphasize one gesture over another, since the client might adopt an exaggerated version of the sound.

13. Remind the client to use the growling dog sound (grrr), the tiger sound (grrr), the growling sound, the arm wresting sound (errr), the middle sound, the flowing sound, or the lifter sound (Lindamood and Lindamood, 1998).

Sound Approximation

1. Shape /ɚ/ from the client's incorrect production. Instruct the client to sustain his error sound and then provide cues for him to reposition the tongue. For example: "Lift your tongue—pull it back a little more—good, hold it—do you hear that?"

2. Shape /ɚ/ from /ʊ/. Ask the client to say the middle sound in "put." Then tell him to prolong that sound. Next instruct him to slowly move his tongue backward. Use a tongue depressor to guide the movement if necessary. When the client produces /ɚ/, have him listen to the new sound. Then have him stop saying it but hold the same tongue position, and then say /ɚ/ without using /ʊ/. Sometimes you will need to have him "turn that new sound on and off" before he can say /ɚ/ spontaneously.

3. Shape /ɚ/ from /ɑ/. Instruct the client to prolong /ɑ/, then slowly raise the tip of his tongue up and back. When /ɑɚ/ is attained, ask him to hold on to the end /ɑɚ/. Use a tongue depressor to guide the movement of the tongue if necessary.

4. Shape /ɚ/ from /ɛ/ Ask the client to say the word "bet," then prolong the vowel /ɛ/ in "bet." Then slowly raise the tongue tip up and back to elicit /ɛɚ/. Instruct him to sustain the end of /ɛɚ/, which is /ɚ/. Guide movement with tongue depressor if necessary.

5. Shape /ɚ/ from /i/. Have the client prolong the /i/ andsimultaneously raise the tongue tip or pull the tongue back, while keeping the sides of the tongue against the upper teeth.

6. Shape /ɚ/ from /r/. Instruct the client to sustain the beginning part of the first sound of the word "run," then hold that sound like a purr.

7. Shape /ɚ/ from /i/. Instruct him to prolong a tense /i/. While the client is saying the /i/, direct him to lift the tongue and curl back the tongue tip to say /ɚ/. An alternate is to ask the client to relax the lips and move the tongue back gradually to produce the /ɚ/.

8. Shape the /ɚ/ from /l/. Tell the client to sustain the /l/ sound while dragging the tip of the tongue slowly back along the roof of the mouth—so far back that you may need to drop the tongue tip slightly. Accompany the directions with hand gestures, such as moving the fingertips back slowly with the palm turned upward. Meanwhile, systematically increase the rate of sequences of /lɚ, lɚ, lɚ/.

9. Shape /ɚ/ from /d/. Instruct the client to place his tongue up and say /d/, then drop the tip of the tongue slightly and say /ɚ/.

10. Shape /ɚ/ from /z/. Tell the client to prolong the /z/ sound, lower the jaw, and pull the tongue back. Also, tell the client to say a hard or quick /z/ with tongue movement backward.

11. Shape /ɚ/ from /ʒ/. Ask the client to hold his tongue in the position for /ʒ/ while you lower his jaw.

12. Shape /ɚ/ from /n/. Instruct the client to spread the sides of his mouth with his fingers and prolong /n/. Then ask him to curl the tip of his tongue backward. As an alternative, instruct the client to sustain a long /n/ while curling the tip of the tongue toward the roof of the mouth to produce the /ɚ/.

13. Shape /ɚ/ from /θ/ or /ð/. Instruct him to prolong /ð/ and then pull the tip of the tongue back quickly and upward toward the alveolar ridge.

14. Shape /ɚ/ from a /t/ and /d/. Practice the sequence /tɚ-dɚ, tɚ-dɚ/. Tell the client to pull his tongue back from /t/ and /d/.

15. Ask children to imitate the purr of a kitten, a growl, or the crow of the rooster.

Chapter 3

Vowel Sounds: Monophthongs

Articulation of Vowels

In contrast to consonants, vowel sounds are produced with the vocal tract relatively open and with no significant constriction between articulators. Vowels are traditionally classified by place of articulation. In English, vowels are voiced under most conditions and nasalized under predictable phonetic conditions. They also serve as the nucleus of most syllables in English. Vowels can be divided into two basic categories: monophthongs and diphthongs. Monophthongs are those vowels which are relatively "steady state" and maintain the same basic articulatory shape and auditory quality throughout their production. The majority of vowels in English can be considered monophthongs. Diphthongs are vowels which move from one articulatory shape (or auditory quality) at vowel onset (the onglide) to another shape at the vowel offset (the offglide). An example in Standard American English is the vowel in the word "hide."

Classification of Vowels (Monophthongs)

The primary articulator used in the production of all vowel sounds is the tongue. The place of articulation refers to the position of the highest point of the tongue in the oral cavity. Tongue position is described in terms of both tongue height and tongue advancement.

Tongue height refers to the relative position of the highest portion of the tongue (high, mid, or low) relative to the roof of the mouth. High vowels such as those found in "heat" (/i/) and "who" (/u/) are produced with the tongue close to the roof of the mouth (and with the lower jaw relatively high). Low vowels, such as those found in "had" (/æ/) and "hot" (/ɑ/), are produced with the tongue much lower in the mouth and with the jaw lowered (and the mouth much more open). Mid vowels, such as those found in "head" (/ɛ/) and "hoe" (/o/), are produced with the tongue somewhere in the middle of the mouth (with the jaw opening somewhere between open and close).

Tongue advancement refers to the relative position of the tongue body (front, central, or back) in the oral cavity as the vowel is produced. Front vowels include those in "heat" (/i/), "hit" (/ɪ/), "hate" (/e/), "head" (/ɛ/), and "hat" (/æ/). However, the high front vowels (e.g., /i/) are produced with the tongue body more forward than for low front vowels (e.g., /æ/). Back vowels are produced with the tongue body pulled back in the oral cavity, such as the vowels in "who" (/u/), "hood" (/ʊ/), "boat" (/o/), "bought" (/ɔ/) and "pot" (/ɑ/). There are few vowels in American English that are produced with the tongue body near the center of the oral cavity. These include the vowels in "but" (/ʌ/) and "bird" (/ɝ/), and the second, unstressed vowels in "data" (/ə/) and "butter" (/ɚ/). The vowel /ʌ/ is sometimes described as being mid and central; however, in most dialects of American English, /ʌ/ is produced somewhat lower and more retracted than /ə/. In contrast, British English uses the mid central vowel /ɜ/ in the word "bird."

Other Characteristics

Three other phonetic features are often used to describe vowel quality: tense/lax, round/nonround, and oral/nasalized.

Tense/Lax

Three pairs of vowels in American English, /i/ / /ɪ/, /e/ /ɛ/, and /u/ /ʊ / are said to differ in terms of "tension," although the phonetic difference between these pairs of vowels are better described in terms of other phonetic features. In particular, the tense vowels /ieu/ are usually longer, higher, and less centralized than their lax counterparts /ɪɛʊ/. In American English phonology, tense vowels can appear in open syllables (syllables ending with a vowel rather than a consonant), as in "he," "hay" and "who"; but lax vowels generally cannot.

Round/Nonround

Lip rounding also affects vowel quality in American English. In particular, the back vowels /u, ʊ, o, ɔ/ all have some degree of lip rounding, with the high vowels usually ittle lip rounding in their normal speech patterns; however, this does not normally affect their intelligibility.

Oral/Nasalized

A final vowel feature is nasalization, which is produced with the velopharyngeal port (the opening between the pharynx and the nasal cavity) open. If a vowel is produced in an open syllable, the speaker normally closes the velopharyngeal port by raising and retracting the velum to the pharyngeal wall. Vowels produced with the velopharyngeal port closed are called "oral vowels," because all of the acoustic energy and air goes through the oral cavity. However, vowels produced in front of a nasal consonant (/m, n, ŋ/) are produced with the velum lowered and the velopharyngeal port open. These vowels are thus "nasalized," as acoustic energy and air passes through both the oral cavity and the nasal cavity. Opening the velopharyngeal port during the production of a vowel imparts a "nasal" quality to the vowel (acoustically, it introduces "nasal formant" and "nasal zeroes" into the vowel spectrum). However, English listeners expect to hear nasalized vowels before nasal consonants and oral vowels in other phonetic contexts; thus, they are relatively unaware of the differences in vowel quality that nasalization produces. However, when vowels are nasalized before non-nasal consonants or in open syllables, English listeners are sensitive to the difference and recognize the speaker's utterance as being "nasal." Excessive nasalization in all phonetic contexts may affect the intelligibility of the speaker.

Table 3.1 describes each vowel in terms of place and manner of articulation, tension, rounding, and stress. The next portions of the chapter describe common errors in vowel articulation and techniques for eliciting vowel production.

Table 3.1 Classification of Vowels

Vowel	Classification
i (beat)	high, front, tense, unrounded
ɪ (bit)	high, front, lax, unrounded
e (bait)	mid, front, tense, unrounded
ɛ (bet)	mid, front, lax, unrounded
æ (bat)	low, front, lax, unrounded
u (boot)	high, back, tense, rounded
ʊ (book)	high, back, lax, rounded
o (boat)	mid, back, tense, rounded
ɔ (bought)	mid-low, back, tense, rounded
ɑ (bomb)	low, back, tense, unrounded
ʌ (but)	mid, central, lax, unrounded
ə (about)	mid, central, lax, unrounded
ɝ murder	mid, central, rounded* (stressed)
ɚ murder	mid, central, rounded* (unstressed)

Most speakers will produce these r-colored vowels with rounding.

/i/

PMV Features:

high/front/tense/
unrounded

Production:

The tongue is raised toward
the palate without making
contact, while the sides of the tongue contact the upper teeth. The lips are
spread, not rounded, and the lips are almost, but not quite, closed.

/ɪ/

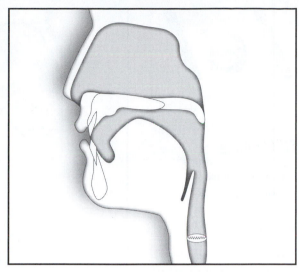

PMV Features:

high/front/tense/
unrounded

Production:

The tongue is raised toward the palate, almost as high as for /i/, while the sides of the tongue contact the upper teeth. The tongue is near the front of the mouth, but more retracted than for /i/. The lips are not rounded and are almost, but not quite, closed.

/e/

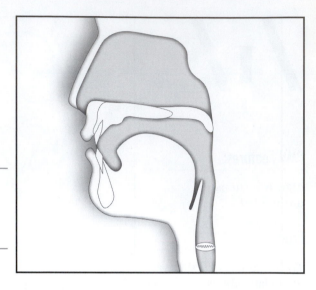

PMV Features:

mid/front/tense/
unrounded

Production:

The front part of the
tongue is raised toward
the palate, slightly below the position for /ɪ/; however, in many speakers the
tongue is more advanced for /e/ than for /ɪ/, although less advanced than for
/i/. In the production of /e/, the sides of the tongue contact the upper teeth.
The lips are not rounded and are almost, but not quite, closed.

/ ɛ /

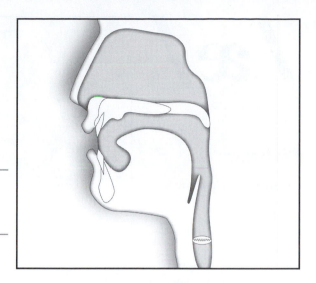

PMV Features:

mid/front/lax/unrounded

Production:

The highest portion of the tongue is raised toward the palate, slightly below the position for /e/, and the tongue body is retracted somewhere behind the position for /e/. The sides of the tongue contact the upper teeth. The lips are not rounded and are open a littler wider than for /ɛ/.

/ æ /

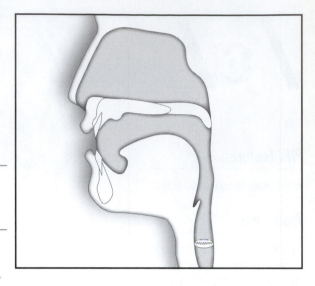

PMV Features:

low/front/lax/unrounded

Production:

The front part of the tongue is raised slightly toward the palate. The jaw is open relatively wide, and the lips are not rounded. Generally, the tongue does not touch the upper teeth during the production of /æ/.

/ u /

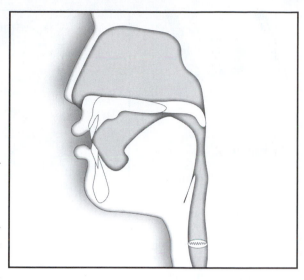

PMV Features:

high/back/tense/rounded

Production:

The back part of the tongue is raised very high toward the palate but does not contact it, and the tongue is retracted toward the velum. The lips are rounded and slightly open.

/ ʊ /

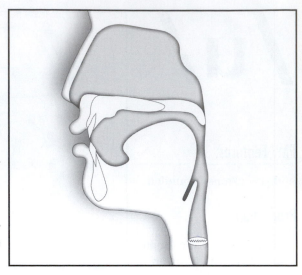

PMV Features:

high/back/lax/rounded

Production:

The back part of the tongue is raised toward the palate, slightly below the position for /u/, but the tongue is somewhat more advanced. The lips are rounded and open slightly.

/o/

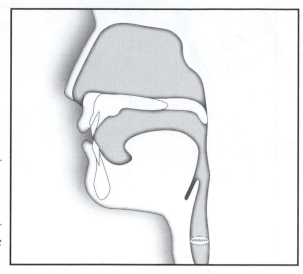

PMV Features:

mid/back/tense/rounded

Production:

The back part of the tongue is lifted halfway to the palate, and the tongue is some- what more retracted than for /ʊ/. The lips are rounded and open slightly.

/ɔ/

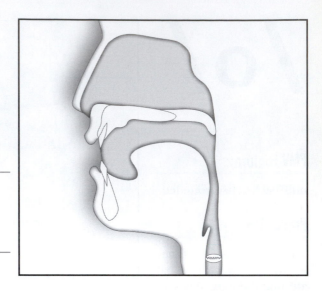

PMV Features:

mid-low/back/tense/
rounded

Production:

The back part of the
tongue is slightly lower
than for /o/, and the tongue tip rests on the floor of the oral cavity. The lips are
slightly rounded, and the mouth is relatively open.

/ɑ/

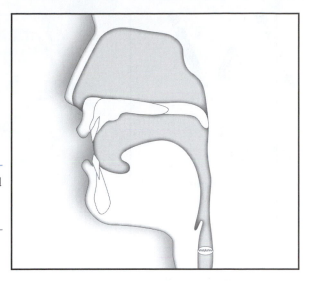

PMV Features:

low/back/tense/unrounded

Production:

The tongue is very low in the mouth, and the jaw is very open. For some speakers, the tongue is very retracted, but it can be relatively central in other speakers, depending on the dialect. The lips are not rounded and are open wide.

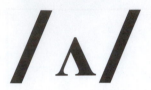

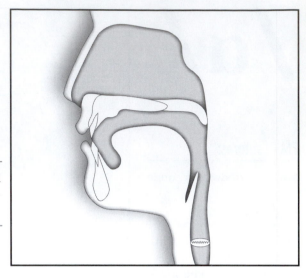

PMV Features:

low/central/lax/unrounded

Production:

The front of the tongue rests on the floor of the oral cavity, while the central part of the tongue is raised slightly toward the palate. The lips are not rounded and are slightly open. This vowel is produced with the tongue lower than the position for the following centralized vowel /ə/.

/ə/

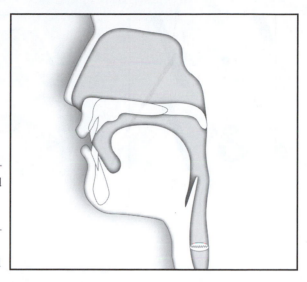

PMV Features:

mid/central/lax/unrounded

Production:

The /ə/ vowel is usually short in duration, produced with the tongue in the middle of the mouth and centralized, with no lip rounding. This vowel is often produced as a reduced phonetic variant of other vowels in unstressed positions. This vowel is often called a "schwa."

/ ɝ /
/ ɚ /

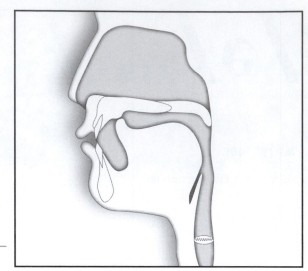

PMV Features:

mid/central/rounded

Production:

These two vowels are produced with the body of the tongue in the same mid central location as for /ə/. The primary phonetic difference between these two vowels and /ə/ is that they are r-colored and often rounded. As we will see in the next chapter, r-colored vowels can be produced in several different ways, including retroflexion (in which the tongue tip is curled back) or "bunched tongue" articulation (the back of the tongue is raised toward the velum). In general, there is little phonetic difference between /ɝ/ and /ɚ/; rather, the difference is one of accepted transcription practice. The symbol /ɝ/ is used when the vowel being transcribed is stressed (as in "b<u>ir</u>d," "m<u>ur</u>der" and "b<u>ur</u>ger"), whereas the symbol /ɚ/ is used when the vowel being transcribed is unstressed (as in "butt<u>er</u>," "murd<u>er</u>" and "burg<u>er</u>"). Both of these vowels can also be considered as "syllabic" versions of the consonant /r/.

Common Contextual Variants

1. **Reduced Vowels:** In short, unstressed syllables, such as the second and fourth syllables in the word "pos<u>si</u>bili<u>ty</u>," the vowels may become "reduced" or "centralized." This means that the vowel is produced less peripherally in the vowel space: the tongue placement for the vowel is closer to the mid central area. In rapid, informal speech, vowels made be reduced completely to /ə/. This phenomenon is also called "vowel neutralization," since there are no evident phonological differences between vowels when they are reduced to schwa.

2. **Voiceless Vowels:** Although vowels are generally voiced, in certain phonetic contexts, a vowel can be partially or even fully devoiced. For example, many people who live in Chicago pronounce their city's name by producing the /i/ in the initial syllable as a voiceless [i̥]. This variation occurs because the syllable is quite short in duration and is preceded and followed by voiceless consonants. Some degree of devoicing is not unexpected in these voiceless phonetic contexts, especially when the vowel is short and reduced.

3. **Omission of Vowels:** In unstressed syllables in rapid, informal speech, speakers often omit vowels: for example, saying "genral" instead of "general" (omitting the second vowel), "polite" as something close to "plight" or "police" as something like "plice." In reality, a very short vowel which has been devoiced (see number 2 above) will often sound as if it has been omitted. However, the normal speaker should be able to produce these vowels in these unstressed positions in slower and more formal speaking situations.

4. **Diphthongization:** The vowels considered thus far have been characterized as being steady-state monophthongs. However, at least two vowels in most dialects of American English, /e/ and /o/, are more commonly produced as the diphthongs [eɪ] and [oʊ], respectively. For example, in the vowel /e/ in the word "bay," the tongue position at the vowel onset is mid-front, but it moves to a higher and more advanced position by the end of the vowel. This vowel would be transcribed phonetically as [eɪ]. Similarly, the vowel /o/ in the word "dough" begins as a mid back rounded vowel, but the tongue rises into the position for a high back rounded vowel by the end of the syllable. The phonetic transcription for this vowel would be [oʊ]. These vowels are often called "non-phonemic diphthongs," since the diphthong as a whole is not phonemically different from its monophthongal counterpart. Other vowels also undergo some diphthongization in syllable-medial and syllable-final position, although in practice, these changes are rarely transcribed. For example, the vowel /ɪ/ often has a centralized offglide ([ɪə]).

Dialectical Variation

Phonetic differences among the various dialects in American English—especially among regional as opposed to social dialects—are most often found in the vowels. For example, in some dialects, the words "pin" and "pen" are produced with two distinct vowels; in other dialects, these two words are homophones. In a dialect common to New York City, speakers make a three-way vowel distinction among the words "merry," "Mary," and "marry." In other dialects, these three words are homophones, or they may exhibit only two different vowel distinctions. The nature and degree of diphthongization in the vowels described thus far also differ from dialect to dialect. For example, in some versions of Appalachian English, the non-phonemic diphthong [eɪ] is more likely to be produced as [ɛɪ]. It is up to the clinician to discover the most common vocalic variations in the client's speech before determining the error patterns in that client's speech. For additional information on dialectal variation in the United States, consult *The Atlas of North American English* (2005) by William Labov, Sharon Ash, and Charles Mouton de Gruyter.

Common Errors

1. **Substitution.** Vowel substitutions are errors involving one or more of the following:

   a.   The height of the tongue in the mouth. For example, the substitution of /ɛ/ (a mid-front vowel) for /ɪ/ (a high front vowel), or the substitution of /ɑ/ (a low back vowel) for /ɔ/ (a low-mid back vowel).

   b.   Incorrect amount of tension in the tongue when a tense vowel such as /i/ is substituted for the lax vowel /ɪ/; or the lax vowel /ɛ/ is substituted for the tense vowel /e/.

   c.   Incorrect tongue placement (the greatest advancement of the tongue, whether it is in the front, middle, or back of the mouth). For example, the substitution of /ɑ/ (a low back vowel) for /æ/ (a low front vowel).

   d.   Inappropriate lip rounding. For example, the substitution of /y/ a (high front rounded vowel not normally found in English) for /i/ (a high front unrounded vowel). As indicated before, speakers vary considerably in their degree of lip rounding for the non-low back vowels.

2. **Neutralization of Vowels.** Neutralization of vowels refers to the production several vowels using an articulatory posture which is at or near that of the neutral vowel /ə/. Neutralization of vowels in unstressed syllables is very common in running speech; but excessive neutralization of vowels is considered non-standard, since it implies a limited repertoire of vowel sounds in the client's phonological system.

3. **Exaggeration of Jaw Movements.** Exaggerated movements of the jaw are very often a cause of incorrect tongue placements and/or abnormal lip positions. Exaggeration can occur as a result of therapy techniques. A speech sound is often taught initially using an exaggerated articulatory posture, which, if not gradually faded out, may remain or even become more exaggerated than before.

4. **Diphthongization of Vowels.** Diphthongization occurs when a steady-state vowel (a monophthong) is pronounced as a diphthong. As noted above, this is not always considered an error production, as in the case of the non-phonemic diphthongs /eɪ/ and /oʊ/ being substituted for the vowels /e/ and /o/, respectively, in stressed syllables. An example of improper diphthongization of a vowel occurs in the English dialect of the Central Ohio region, where sometimes the word "at" is pronounced [æət] instead of /æt/.

5. **Excessive or Inappropriate Nasalization of Vowels.** Excessive and/or inappropriate nasalization of vowels across a wide range of phonetic contexts (especially when the vowel is not followed by a nasal consonant) is a result of insufficient velopharyngeal closure.

6. **Omission of Vowels.** The omission of the unstressed vowel, especially if it has been reduced to schwa, is a common occurrence and not always abnormal. However, if the client consistently omits vowels, especially in stressed positions, the clinician should investigate further.

Eliciting Techniques

In the absence of imitation or a facilitating context, the following strategies may be used.

Phonetic Placement

In vowel placement, the speaker can manipulate four variables: the height of the tongue, the placement of the tongue in the mouth, the amount of tension in the tongue, and the amount of lip rounding. Show correct articulatory posture to the client using pictures, mirrors, therapist demonstrations, and direct manipulation of the client's tongue with a tongue depressor. Taction may also be useful for eliciting a particular vowel sound. For example, instruct the client to place his index finger on clinician's tongue as she produces and maintains the sound. The client then places his other index finger on his tongue to imitate the correct tongue position. The tension in the tongue may be increased by having the client produce the lax vowel of a tense-lax pair while clinician places her fingers on either side of the client's lower jaw. Press inward on the jaw firmly to increase tension in the tongue.

Proprioceptive Feedback

1. Contrasting the features of the vowels while emphasizing the propriocep-
   tive feedback (i.e., feeling the posture of the articulators) assists the client
   in eliciting vowel production. Suggested contrasts include the following:

   a. Tongue position:
      1) Front-central-back
      2) High-mid-low (roof/top of mouth, floor/bottom of mouth; mid-
         level, up-down)

   b. Jaw position (the jaw/chin posture is closely related to the tongue
      posture):
      1) Lowered (dropped, down)-raised (up, high)
      2) Open (wide)-closed

   c. Lip posture (how does the outside of the mouth look?):
      1) Smiling (spread; slightly parted; corners of the mouth are
         pulled back)
      2) Oval (yawn)
      3) Rounded (protruded)

   d. Tension of lips, tongue and jaw
      1) Lax (relaxed)-tense

   e. Tongue movement
      1) Simple-glided

2. Lindamood (1998) suggests the following labels for the vowels to emphasize the shape of the mouth:

   > *Smiles (front vowels)*
   > *Opens (central vowels)*
   > *Rounds (back vowels)*
   > *Sliders (diphthongs)*

Lindamood also suggests using imagery by referring to the jaw and tongue posturing as moving up and down stairs or moving from the front to back stairs. The
client is instructed to move the chin and tongue from the top to the bottom of
the stairs depending on the posture of the specific vowel. Adjacent vowels on
the vowel quadrant are thought of as moving in "little steps" versus "big jumps."

Successive Approximation

In the successive approximation technique, the client produces the error
sound and is instructed on subsequent trials to lower or raise the tongue
slightly and/or to make the lips rounder or less round until correct production
of the target vowel is achieved. For example, if the client produces /i/ for /e/,
he is instructed to try again with his tongue slightly lower in his mouth, until
the /e/ sound is produced.

Sound Approximation

Prolongation of a vowel can sometimes help elicit the target vowel. The vowel /e/ will often cause the client to produce /i/, especially if the client is producing the diphthong [eɪ]. In addition, prolonging the vowel /õ/, especially in the diphthong [oʊ], will often elicit the vowel /u/. The clinician can also instruct the client to produce a vowel, the tongue placement of which is slightly above or below the target vowel, and then ask the client to lower or raise the tongue to the position of a vowel either below or above the target vowel. For example, for the vowel /e/, the client is told to produce /ɛ/ and then to slowly raise his tongue until he produces the vowel /i/. Before he reaches the tongue height necessary for /i/, he will have produced the target vowel /e/.

Moto-Kinesthetic Techniques

/i/

Using latex gloves, the clinician moves the client's lower jaw downward slightly so that the incisors show. The thumb and forefinger of one hand are placed on the client's upper lip, each about an inch apart from the midline. Pressure is exerted there. The thumb and forefinger of the other hand are placed similarly under the lower lip, but no pressure is exerted.

/ɪ/

The jaw is lowered a little more than for /i/. Stimulate outside by drawing the upper lip more toward the corners and touching the middle area of the lower lip with the end of a tongue depressor. Stimulate inside using the end of a tongue depressor to dip the end of the tongue.

/e/ and /eɪ/

Set the mouth at a position slightly above that for /æ/. Place the thumb and forefinger on the lower jaw about halfway from the midline to the corners. Place the thumb and forefinger of the other hand on the upper lip in the position for /i/. Provide an auditory model of /eɪ/ and simultaneously raise the jaw upward moving both lips to the corners, toward /i/.

/ɛ/

Bring the jaw down slightly more than for /i/. The lips are drawn to the corners. Stimulate outside by applying pressure with your index finger to the midline just below the lower lip. If this fails, stimulate inside by pressing the two sides of the end of the tongue together toward the midline with two halves of a tongue depressor.

/æ/

For an outside stimulation, the jaw is lowered slightly more than for /ɛ/. The upper lip is held by the thumb and forefinger of one hand. Place the thumb and forefinger of the other hand at equal distances from the midline of the lower lip, and exert pressure against the jaw outward from the midline. Stimulate inside by placing the flat surface of a tongue depressor on the edges of the lower teeth, about three-quarters of an inch from the end of the depressor. The surface of the tongue depressor inside the mouth serves to shape the tongue like an inclined plane, sloping toward the tip.

/ʌ/ and /ə/

The jaw is slightly more closed than for /æ/ and the tongue is retracted more toward the central position. No additional muscular activity is stimulated.

/u/

The thumb and forefinger of one hand are placed toward the corners of the client's lip while the lower lip is held similarly with the other hand. The lips are moved together toward the center to create the round shape for /u/.

/ʊ/

Same as that for /u/ except the lips are moved inward for rounding and then outward in a "scooplike" position to attain a more relaxed lip posture.

/o/ or /oʊ/

Set the mouth in the position for /ɑ/. Provide an auditory model and use both hands to move the areas above and below the lips outward and toward the center until the position for /u/ is reached.

/ɔ/

With one hand, move the jaw downward but not as far as for /ɑ/ (on the following page). Place the thumb and forefinger of one hand at points halfway between the midline and the corners of the mouth below the lower lip. Place the thumb and forefinger of the other hand at the corners of the throat, as in the stimulation for /k/. Press the lips slightly toward the middle and outward.

/ɑ/

The thumb and forefinger of one hand are placed on the client's upper lip at an equal distance from the midline. The thumb and forefinger of the other hand are placed at points halfway between the midline and the corners of the mouth below the lower lip. Pressure is exerted inward while the lower jaw is brought downward, slightly lower than for /ɔ/.

Chapter 4

Vowel Sounds: Diphthongs

Classification of Vowels (Diphthongs)

A combination of two vowels in the same syllable is called a *diphthong*. There are three traditional phonemic diphthongs in American English: /aɪ/, /aʊ/, and /ɔɪ/. As opposed to non-phonemic diphthongs (like [eɪ], the on-glide for a phonemic diphthong is phonologically distinct from the diphthong itself. For example, /ɔɪ/ (as in "soy") is a distinct phoneme from /ɔ/ (as in "saw"). This chapter also covers a fourth diphthong—/ju/ as in *use* and *few*. However, there is some disagreement as to whether /ju/ should be considered a true diphthong or simply as a glide + vowel combination. For example, Ladefoged (2001) presents /ju/ as a diphthong, whereas Catford (1988) does not, since phoneticians normally do not view other /j/ + vowel combinations (such as /jɛs/ in "yes") as examples of a diphthong.

Diphthongs are produced when two vowel sounds are produced as a glide. Their phonetic transcription shows the two vowels combined. For example, the /ɔɪ/ in "boy" shows the symbols for the two vowel sounds /ɔ/ and /ɪ/. Thus, the sound /ɔɪ/ is produced by rapid movements beginning at the position for /ɔ/ (the onglide) and ending at the position for /ɪ/ (the offglide). To feel this movement, you have only to produce the sound slowly. In so doing, you may well overshoot the terminal sound and produce the sound /i/. In contrast, in rapid speech, we have a tendency to undershoot the /ɪ/. However, the resulting sound can still be identified as the single unit /ɔɪ/. The same pattern holds true for the other non-phonemic diphthongs.

Figure 4.1 diagrams the direction of movement in the three traditional diphthongs and /ju/. Note that the three traditional diphthongs are all produced with a rising movement of the tongue, and they are often called rising diphthongs. The diphthong /ju/ is produced by movement from a high-front position to a high-back position.

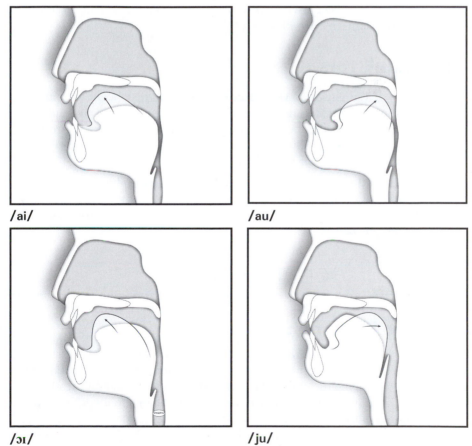

/ai/

/au/

/ɔɪ/

/ju/

Figure 4.1 Production of four phonemic diphthongs

Common Contextual Variants

Diphthongs can undergo the same types of contextual variation, including devoicing and nasalization, as do the monophthongs. Diphthongs can also undergo monophthongization—that is, the diphthong is produced as a monophthong, but usually only the onglide is produced.

Dialectical Variation

There are phonetic differences among the various dialects in American English, especially among regional as opposed to social dialects. These differences are most often found in the vowels and can extend to the diphthongs. Perhaps the most commonly recognized differences across dialects are variations in the production of the diphthong /aɪ/. In many Appalachian dialects, the diphthong /aɪ/ is produced as the monophthong /ɑ/. In other dialects, the diphthong /aɪ/ may be produced with a different onglide (as in /ɔɪ/) or offglide (as in /aə/). Again, the clinician must be aware of the vocalic differences between the client's dialect (whether it be a regional or social dialect) and that of so-called Standard American English.

Common Errors

1. **Absence of Transitional Movements.** The client may begin with an articulatory posture at or near that of the first component of the diphthong but he fails to complete the transitional movements necessary to produce the second component sound of the diphthong. For example, the client may produce *out* as /at/ rather than /aʊt/.

2. **Faulty Initiation of the Diphthong.** The client may initiate the diphthong with an incorrect articulatory posture. When this happens, a word such as *kite* may be produced as /keɪt/, rather than /kaɪt/, or the word *oil* as /əɪl/, rather than as /ɔɪl/.

Eliciting Techniques

Phonetic Placement

The clinician explains the movements necessary to produce the diphthong to the client using diagrams, a mirror, and demonstration. The use of taction may be beneficial by having the client place his (latex gloved) hand on the clinician's jaw to sense its posture or place his hand on the lips to identify openness (rounding) of the lips.

Successive Approximation

Successive approximation is used to gradually modify the client's articulation error. The client is instructed to begin by producing her error sound. He is then asked to repeat it but is given a series of instructions, such as "raise or lower the tongue slightly," or "don't round your lips so much," or "round your lips more," until the correct production is attained. For example, if the client produces /eɪ/ for /ɔɪ/, he should be instructed to try again rounding the lips a little more. He can then be instructed to try again with his lips rounded but with his tongue slightly lower and farther back in the mouth. Repeat these instructions until correct production of /ɔɪ/ is achieved.

Moto-Kinesthetic

Phonemic Diphthongs

/aɪ/

/aɪ/ is composed of /a/ and /ɪ/.[1] Thus, set the client's jaw in the position for /a/ and then move directly upward to the position for /ɪ/, moving the lips toward the corners.

/aʊ/

/aʊ/ is composed of an onglide slightly more advanced than /ɑ/ and /ʊ/. Bring the client's lower jaw down for /ɑ/. Use auditory stimulation: with both hands, move the areas above and below the lips outward toward the center, as necessary for /ʊ/.

/ɔɪ/

/ɔɪ/ is composed of /ɔ/ and /ɪ/. Set the client's mouth in the position for /ɔɪ/. Then move the lips away from the midline toward the position for /ɪ/.

/ju/

/ju/ is composed of /j/ and /u/. Set the client's mouth to the position for /i/ and stimulate /i/. Move your thumb and forefinger from the corners of the upper lip toward the center into the position for /u/.

---

[1] Although the two symbols /a/ and /ɑ/ are two distinct phonetic segments, they are essentially similar when describing the two rising diphthongs /aɪ/ and /aʊ/. The phoneme /a/ is slightly more forward than /ɑ/, but both are described as low-back vowels. The two symbols /a/ and /ɑ/ can be used interchangeably when representing onglide of the diphthongs /aɪ/ and /aʊ/.

Chapter 5

/r/ and /ɚ/ From Science to Practice

This chapter concentrates on the "r" sound, because it is responsible for perhaps the greatest amount of clinical frustration of all the sounds of American English. A major reason for this frustration is that the basic acoustic and physiological science of /r/—both the prevocalic and postvocalic variants—has not been well understood until recently. As a result, the science behind the techniques used in the clinic has not been explained to clinicians in a way that clinicians can use.

The purpose of this chapter is to fill this gap in clinician knowledge, by showing how recent developments in our scientific understanding can improve the use of techniques discussed in this book. The first section of this chapter discusses in detail current knowledge regarding /r/ phonetics and articulation. In particular, it addresses the question of why /r/ is particularly difficult for language learners and teachers. A substantial portion of this discussion examines the scientific basis of the traditional distinction between prevocalic, or consonantal, /r/ and the postvocalic, "syllabic," or "vocalic" /r/ (often written with the /ɚ/ symbol).

The second section explains the interaction between this knowledge and the teaching techniques discussed earlier in the book—in other words, the interaction of theory and practice. Note that in all cases, unless there is a specific need to refer to the prevocalic versus postvocalic distinction, the "r" sound will be referred to phonetically as /r/.

Overall, the important message of this chapter is fourfold:

1. American English speakers produce /r/ in a number of ways. The diversity of ways to produce /r/ matches the diversity of techniques that work for teaching it.

2. Some tongue shapes may not work for some vocal tracts. What works to produce a correct-sounding /r/ for one client may not work for another.

3. A clinician may need to experiment in order to match tongue configurations to a particular client, especially in cases of "resistant" /r/ (Clark et al., 1993).

4. Such "custom design" requires an understanding of the fundamental factors involved in producing acceptable American English /r/.

Scientific Issues in /r/ Phonetics

Definitions of Symbols and Targets

The description and categorization of /r/ articulation in Chapter 2 and in this chapter corresponds to the definition given in many standard textbooks. Similarly, the symbols for /r/ sounds used in Chapter 2 and in this chapter follow the common conventions of treating the /r/ phonemes used in pre- and postvocalic syllable position and in stressed versus unstressed environments as separate entities (/r/, /ɚ/, /ɝ/). As explained later in the chapter, these conventional characterizations are used in speech-language pathology largely for historical and practical purposes. In reality, these two symbols reflect the same tongue shapes produced with different articulatory timing. As a result, this chapter uses the symbol /ɚ/ only rarely, when the history of its use is discussed in detail. The /r/ will be used in all other cases.

It is important to distinguish between /r/ as a target vocal tract shape achieved by the articulatory system during speech (i.e., as a phoneme) and as the goal of a therapy session, which may be described in more simplistic terms that make sense to the client. A potentially confusing aspect of the clinical literature is the use of phrases such as "the 21 ways to say /r/" (Ristuccia et al., 2004). These phrases make reference to the practical fact that a clinician may wish to use different techniques for teaching /r/ in different phonetic and prosodic contexts. These multiple techniques exist because a client who has learned a sound under one set of coarticulatory demands may have trouble accommodating to a different set of coarticulatory demands. Difficulty with coarticulation is particularly likely to occur when /r/ is combined with different vowels, because the production of /r/ and adjacent vowels overlaps in time. Accordingly, a client may require specific and detailed training for each separate combination. Similarly, there are reasons why clinicians have found it helpful to consider pre- and postvocalic /r/, or stressed versus unstressed /r/, as separate entities for training purposes. Nevertheless, the practical necessity of training for different conditions in some clients does not mean that there are 21 separate linguistic allophones of /r/. As discussed below, in most cases, vowels and /r/ combine in predictable ways. Similarly, /r/ combines with word stress, or with a particular word position, in ways that are predictable from the way prosodic conditions affect the client's sounds. In this chapter, all references to types or varieties of /r/, such as those shown in Figure 5.1, indicate different vocal tract shapes for the /r/ phoneme, rather than different ways to organize its teaching.

Why is /r/ Difficult?

The sound /r/ is difficult for several reasons. The main reason is that the standard American English /r/ has particularly complex articulation, using multiple parts of the tongue plus other articulators. This complexity is displayed in Figure 5.1, which shows midsagittal images of 12 normal healthy native speakers of American English producing sustained /r/.

However, additional factors come into play. These are listed here in order of complexity:

1. Multiple places of articulation along the vocal tract (front-to-back)
2. Precise positioning of sides of tongue

Figure 5.1 Midsagittal MRIs of sustained productions of /r/ by 12 American English speakers. Subjects were directed to sustain the final sound of "pour." (Note that /r/ in postvocalic position is often written with /ɚ/ symbol.) Subjects show a continuum of vocal tract shapes for /r/. The left column shows variants that might fit the standard category of "bunched" /r/. The middle column shows variants that might fit the category of "retroflex." The right column shows variants that involve some combination of the classic "bunched" and "retroflex" shapes. Note, however, that the binary classification into "retroflex" and "bunched" is not sufficient to classify all tongue shapes; for instance, Speaker 10's production might be classified as retroflex, while speaker 11 has some bunching. Similar vocal tract shapes have been recorded dynamically in prevocalic conditions. (These images are reproduced from an ongoing research study sponsored by the U.S. National Institute of Deafness and Other Communication Disorders (R01 DC 005250, P.I. Suzanne Boyce).)

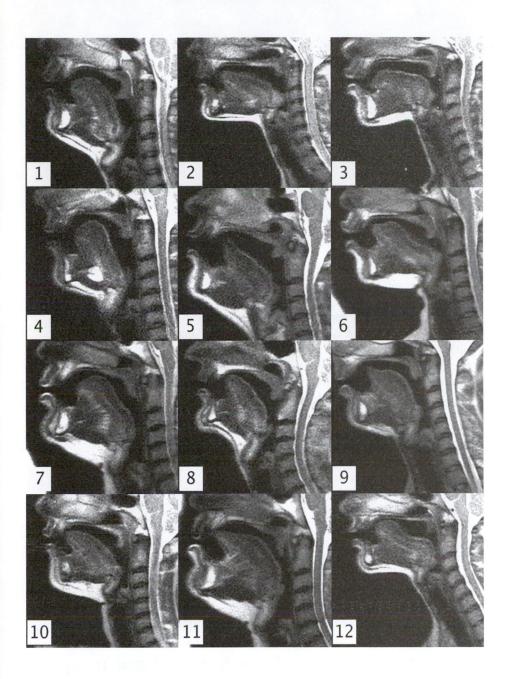

3. Lack of tactile feedback

4. Variability across syllable position and phonetic contexts

5. Variability across speakers and dialects

6. Lack of acoustic specificity for tongue shape

Multiple Places of Articulation

Most sounds require that only one articulator (such as the lips,[1] the tongue dorsum, or the tongue tip) produce a constriction in the vocal tract. Thus, only one articulator must be positioned precisely. Some sounds, such as /w/, require two articulators to be positioned precisely. The three most difficult sounds of English, /s/, /l/, and /r/, require precise front-to-back positioning of a minimum of two articulators for the purpose of making a constriction. For /l/, the two articulators are the tongue tip and the tongue dorsum. For /s/, the two articulators are the tongue tip and tongue blade, both of which must be at a particular distance from the palate.

However, for /r/, the two articulators are variable, depending on the type of /r/ involved. For most types of /r/, the first articulator is the tongue root, which makes a pharyngeal constriction toward the back wall of the pharynx. Depending on the type of /r/ used, the second articulator may be the tongue tip, tongue blade, or tongue dorsum. In addition, some speakers use an /r/ in which both tongue blade and tongue tip, or tongue dorsum and tongue blade, or all three, appear to be precisely positioned to form constrictions. Thus, minimum articulatory precision for /r/ requires correct positioning of two points along the tongue, but many speakers use three.

Rounding also accompanies production of /r/ sounds for many speakers, especially in prevocalic position. Phonologically, rounding is considered to be optional in English—that is, speakers may round as much or as little as they wish during /r/ as long as the resulting sound is recognizable (Stevens and Keyser, 1989). Articulatorily, however, even with adequate tongue shape, some speakers cannot achieve a correct-sounding /r/ without rounding. These speakers can achieve /r/ only by adding a simultaneous lip constriction to their constrictions in the pharynx and along the palate. Thus, if a speaker uses lip rounding, the articulatory complexity of /r/ production is increased; that is, the requirement for a lip constriction of a certain size and shape, in addition to precise placement of two or three points along the tongue from front to back.

Precise Positioning of the Sides of the Tongue

An additional source of complexity for /r/ sounds comes the fact that, like /l/ and /s/, /r/ requires precise positioning of the sides of the tongue. For /l/, the sides of the tongue must angle down, so as to allow the lateral passage of air. For /s/,

---

[1] For this description, the upper lip and lower lip together form a single articulator. Appropriate jaw position is also assumed.

the sides of the tongue must be positioned so as to create a midline groove that narrows and concentrates the airstream. For /r/, the sides of the tongue are positioned differently depending on the type of /r/. Thus, instructions to a client may be different depending on which type of /r/ is being taught. As noted in earlier chapters, in the palatal regions, "retroflex" types of /r/ show a midline groove in the tongue blade, while "bunched" types have a flatter profile in across the lateral surface of the tongue at this point. Recent MRI data has shown that both types of /r/ tongue shapes have some degree of grooving in the tongue dorsum/root area, meaning that the sides of the tongue are angled up in this region. Thus, for all types of /r/, the subject must have good control of the sides of the tongue; and for some types of /r/, the tongue sides may be flat in the region of the tongue blade but raised in the region of the tongue dorsum/root. Note that the images in Figure 5.1 show the shape of the tongue in the midsagittal orientation. In other words, they show the shape of the tongue at the deepest point of the midline groove.

Summary of Precise Positioning Requirements

In essence, to produce a good /r/, speakers must *at a minimum* be able to position at least two points along the tongue with precision. In addition, they must be able to accurately position the sides of the tongue. Speakers who use more complicated types of /r/ must be able to position three points along the tongue with precision. Those speakers who also round their lips add another articulatory requirement to the total. It may be fairly said that the production of even the simplest form of American English /r/ requires a high level of motor skill.

Lack of Tactile Feedback

As noted above, the three most difficult sounds of English, /r/, /s/, and /l/, specify the positioning of the sides of the tongue. For /s/ especially, the sides of the tongue are used as a kind of scaffolding to brace the tongue so that it can stay in place (Stone, 1995). In the case of /s/ and /l/, this positioning is aided by tactile feedback from bracing the tongue against the sides of the teeth. For /r/, however, there is no such use of the teeth for bracing. For some /r/ tongue shapes, there is some tactile feedback: for example, it is possible to feel the tongue lightly touch the molar and pre-molar teeth. This tactile feedback can be used and even exaggerated to direct a client in tongue placement for some "bunched" types of /r/. However, the amount of tactile feedback is highly variable across speakers and tongue shapes. In general, speakers of American English who have learned to produce "correct" /r/ have had to do so with a minimum of tactile feedback. Speakers in search of an acceptable way to produce /r/ are forced to rely largely on acoustic feedback.

Variability According to Syllabic Position and Phonetic Context

To understand the issue of /r/ production, clinicians may find it helpful to understand the history of use of phonetic symbols in describing American English. Among speech pathologists and many linguistic phoneticians, it is traditional to use different symbols for pre- and postvocalic /r/. In prevocalic position, the symbol used is that for "consonantal" /r/. In postvocalic or syllabic positions, the symbol often used is /ɚ/, or "schwar." This transcription tradition acknowledges the fact that /r/ can act both as a consonant and as the nucleus of a syllable. It also recognizes the fact that clients are not evenly successful at producing /r/ in different syllable positions. It also reflects the fact that English dialects can be divided into two groups depending on how they treat postvocalic /r/: "rhotic" and "non-rhotic" (also known in American dialectology as "r-less") dialects.

In the rhotic dialects, pre- and postvocalic /r/'s both sound strongly r-like. In these dialects, a strict phonemic analysis requires that the second syllable of a word like "mother" be transcribed as schwa plus /r/ (Trager and Bloch). However, in postvocalic position the two sounds /ə/ and /r/ are so tightly coarticulated that it is hard to separate their articulation even when speaking very slowly. This means that it is possible to hear them as a single sound /ɚ/. In the non-rhotic dialects (e.g., American East Coast rural [Maine] and urban [Boston], American Southern, British RP), postvocalic /r/ appears to be reduced to a schwa, although some remnants of /r/ may color the quality of the vowel (e.g., Boston [paək] "park," Southern [fajə] "fire"). In American dialects, the degree of r-coloring may range from very noticeable to very minor. In British English non-rhotic dialects postvocalic /r/ is reduced simply to schwa—to the extent that the filler word spelled as "uh" in American English is pronounced with a schwa and spelled "er." In American dialects especially, when following a stressed vowel, the reduced and softened /r/ may be heard less as a schwa, and more as extra lengthening on the vowel (e.g., [faɑ] for "fire" or [paɑk] for "park"). Depending on whether the final syllable of a word like "mother" was analyzed as schwa plus /r/, or a single sound target combining the two, the parallels between postvocalic /r/'s in the rhotic versus non-rhotic dialects were expressed as /ər/ (rhotic) versus /ə/ (non-rhotic), or /ɚ/ (rhotic) versus /ə/ (non-rhotic). For both dialects, the prevocalic /r/ was written as /r/. The schwar symbols of /ɝ/ and /ɚ/ were originally used to indicated the slightly different vowel qualities of schwa followed by /r/ under stressed and unstressed postvocalic conditions.

Historically, the prestige dialect of North America in the early twentieth century was non-rhotic. At about the time of the Second World War, the prestige standard American English dialect changed. However, the change was gradual; and the symbols /ɚ/ and /ɝ/ continued to be used to describe variations in usage. Currently, the prestige standard dialect is "rhotic." In the "rhotic" dialects, /r/ is produced strongly enough to sound like a clear /r/ in all syllable positions. It is generally agreed among linguistic phoneticians that for the current rhotic dialects, pre- and postvocalic /r/'s sound so similar that they may as well be represented by /r/ alone, or as /r/ and /ər/, or as /r/ and /r̩/ (with a syllabic diacritic), as by /r/ and schwar /ɚ/. In other words, for rhotic dialects, the use of two different phonetic symbols does not mean that pre- and postvocalic /r/ constitute different phonemes, or even that they have different articulatory targets. However, as discussed below, the distinction can still be useful in teaching /r/, even for rhotic dialects. In general, most clinicians find themselves aiming for a rhotic dialect in training the pronunciation of their clients.

Articulation of Pre- and Postvocalic /r/ in Rhotic Dialects

As noted above, it is traditional to use different symbols for pre- and postvocalic /r/'s in "rhotic" dialects, even though they belong to the same phoneme. Some researchers have shown data indicating slightly different tongue shapes for /r/ in different syllable positions. For instance, Zawadski and Kuehn (1980) and Shriberg and Kent (1982) found slight differences in the shape of the tongue for speech filmed by X-ray at one hundred frames per second. Similarly, Alwan et al. (1997) asked subjects to hold their tongue position in prevocalic position (at the beginning of a word) or postvocalic position (at the end of a word) for approximately 13 seconds while MRI data was collected, and found slight differences in images of tongue shape. These data have sometimes been interpreted as meaning that speakers aim to reach different phonological or phonetic targets in the different syllable positions. However, the differences noted in these data are very minor when compared to the differences across subjects shown in Figures 5.2a, 5.2b, and 5.3; and they can easily be explained as reflecting uncertainties in the imaging techniques used. In particular, both the X-ray technique used by Zawadski and Kuehn (1980) and Shriberg and Kent (1982), and the MRI technique used by Alwan et al. (1997) effectively compare "snapshots," or "freeze-frames," of tongue motion. An identical movement will look slightly different if imaged at different points in the movement trajectory. Thus, differences in tongue configuration during pre- or postvocalic /r/ may simply reflect a comparison between the same motions "frozen" at slightly different points in time. It is safe to say that there is no substantial evidence that speakers of rhotic dialects have different vocal tract targets for /r/ versus /ɚ/.

Timing of Different Articulations According to Syllabic or Syllable Position

What does seem to differ between pre- and postvocalic /r/ is the way the different constrictions along the vocal tract (i.e., lips, pharynx, tongue-to-palate) are timed with respect to each other (Gick et al., 2006; Browman and Goldstein, 1992). In other words, for normal-sounding adults, articulators for a single sound do not always operate in lockstep but with slightly different patterns of timing movement. New methods of imaging tongue motion have shown that for prevocalic /r/'s, constrictions of the tongue tip/blade are timed to occur simultaneously, such that the tongue, jaw, and lip movements toward constriction all reach their target at the same time. In contrast, for postvocalic /r/'s, the tongue root begins to move toward constriction before the tongue tip/blade begins to move (Gick et al., 2006), and the tongue root movement reaches its target while the tongue tip/blade is still moving. In other words, "rhotic" /r/'s in prevocalic and postvocalic position are produced with the same movement targets, but with different timing. Figures 5.2a and 2b show this difference in tongue root/dorsum versus tongue tip/blade timing for a prevocalic case, where /r/ is syllabified with the following vowel. Overall, the tendency for earlier tongue root/dorsum timing in postvocalic position is a general pattern of American English. Similar patterns have been found for other consonants, including nasals and /l/ (Sproat and Fujimura, 1993; Browman and Goldstein, 1992; Krakow, 1999; Gick et al., 2006).[2]

At present, clinical training techniques for /r/ in pre- and postvocalic positions do not make explicit reference to patterns of timing in articulatory movements. It is hard to imagine saying to a child: "Move your tongue root a tenth of a second before your tongue tip." However, this timing information does explain why it is sometimes important to teach pre- and postvocalic /r/ at separate points in therapy. It makes sense that children and/or English-learning adults might learn a single pattern of articulatory coordination successfully but have difficulty switching to a different pattern in a different prosodic environment.

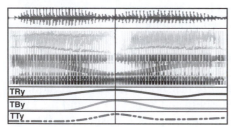

Figure 5.2a Waveform, spectrogram, and superior/inferior (y) transducer position for Tongue Tip (TT), Tongue Body (TB), and Tongue Root (TR) tracked by an electromagnetic magnetometer system (EMMA) during production of the nonsense word /wɑrɑv/. The speaker was a normal adult male speaker of a "rhotic" variety of American English. Notice that the Tongue Root (TRy) movement begins earlier and achieves maximum sooner than that for the Tongue Body (TBy) or Tongue Tip (TTy). (Adapted from Tiede et al., 2006.)

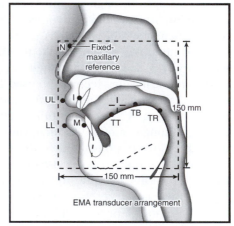

Figure 5.2b Transducer attachment locations on the tongue during RESTING position (not speech). (Adapted from Tiede et al., 2006.)

---

[2] The same researchers have also noted a tendency for tip/blade movements to be less extensive (i.e., weaker) in postvocalic position. The movement target remains the same. For /r/, this tendency is slight in the case of "rhotic" dialects and more extreme in the case of "r-less" dialects. When tip/blade movements are sufficiently attenuated, the result sounds like a schwa. The timing of lip constriction tends to follow tip/blade constriction. This fact explains the often-noted finding that acoustic patterns for /r/, especially the lowering of the third formant, are more pronounced in prevocalic position (Delattre and Freeman, 1968).

As noted later on in the chapter, many of the commonly used elicitation techniques listed in Chapter 2 actually have the effect of encouraging particular timing patterns. For instance, the technique advocated by Garbutt and Arden, and described in Chapter 2, of labeling /r/ in one environment as a "running" /r/ and in another environment as a "standing" /r/ seems in many ways to be an insightful description of the difference in patterns of articulatory timing for pre- and postvocalic or syllabic /r/. Similarly, because /ɑ/ involves a constriction of the tongue root in the pharynx, a technique which shapes /r/ from an initial /ɑ/ may have the effect of encouraging the client to make a tongue root constriction before a tip/blade constriction. Accordingly, the technique of starting from /ɑ/ is likely to be particularly effective in producing postvocalic /r/ timing patterns. It is very likely that although clinicians may not be thinking in these terms, many who are most successful at teaching /r/ have used /r/ elicitation techniques in just this way to encourage change in timing patterns across syllable position.

Articulation of /r/ across Different Phonetic Contexts

Most speakers of American English rhotic dialects do not change tongue shapes according to phonetic context. However, some speakers do seem to switch under some circumstances. As noted above, the bunched and retroflex tongue shapes shown in Figure 5.2a result from different phonetic contexts but are produced by the same speaker (Kent, personal communication). In a study of eight speakers, Guenther et al. (1999) found that seven used the same tongue shape for /dr/, /gr/, and /vr/ clusters, while one speaker used a "bunched" shape for a /gr/ cluster but a "retroflex" shape for all other contexts. Figure 5.3 shows an example of a speaker (speaker 5 in Figure 5.1) with a similar pattern of switching /r/ shapes. Tiede et al. (2005) found that some speakers switch tongue shapes in different /i/, /u/, and /ɑ/ vowel contexts. The factors that lead a speaker to switch tongue shapes are not well understood at this time. However, if a client has more trouble with /r/ in particular phonetic contexts, it is often helpful to use a teaching technique aimed at eliciting a different tongue shape.

Other Clinical Use of the Distinction between "Vocalic" /ɚ/ and "Consonantal" /r/

The difference between pre- and postvocalic /r/ is similar to that between "syllabic" or "vocalic" /r/ and "consonantal" /r/. Ultrasound and other articulatory tracking techniques have shown that speakers normally maintain the same tongue shape for "vocalic" and "consonantal" /r/. However, sometimes a client is successful at producing /r/ as the nucleus of a syllable—i.e., as "vocalic" or "syllabic" /r/—but is less successful when producing /r/ in the prevocalic position. As noted above, the timing pattern of prevocalic /r/ involves simultaneous movement of two separate areas of the tongue—the root and the tongue tip or blade. Similarly, in a sustained "vocalic" /r/, the two areas of the tongue are both in position for constriction in the

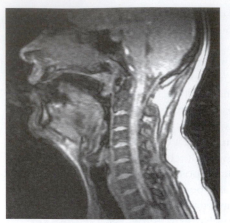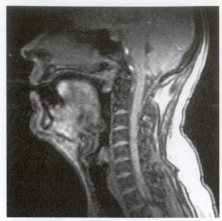

Figure 5.3 MRIs of /r/ produced by speaker 5 of Figure 5.1 during intervocalic /dr/ and /gr/ clusters of the nonsense words /wadrɑv/ and /wagrɑv/ with final stress. The MRI is somewhat fuzzy because of tongue movement during image capture, but the difference in tongue shape is clear. For this speaker, tongue shape is classically retroflex in most environments but alters to a more bunched configuration when following a velar consonant. Data from a speaker with a similar pattern is discussed in Guenther et al. (1999). Some speakers also show changes in tongue shape according to vowel context (Tiede et al., 2005). Other speakers show little or no change in tongue shape across context (Guenther et al., 1999; Tiede et al., 2005). (Images acquired with the help of Kiyoshi Honda, Ph.D., at ATR Laboratories in Japan for an ongoing research study sponsored by the U.S. National Institute of Deafness and Other Communication Disorders (R01 DC 005250, P.I. Suzanne Boyce).)

palatal and pharyngeal regions. Chapter 2 presents a technique that trains the client to produce /rɑ/ by gradually shifting from "vocalic" or "syllabic" /r/ to "consonantal" /r/ (written as /ɚrɑ/, or /r̩rɑ/). This technique works well because the client is being trained to start with the palatal constriction and the pharyngeal constriction already in place. In other words, the client is being trained to start "consonantal" /r/ with the consonantal timing pattern of simultaneous constriction at the palatal and the pharynx.

Variability across Speakers and Alternate Tongue Positions for /r/ and /ɚ/

The most important feature of /r/ is the multiplicity of tongue shapes used by native speakers of American English. Many textbooks give only one description of the articulation of /r/, thereby implying that all speakers use the same tongue configurations for /r/. Some textbooks describe two possible tongue shapes but still imply that these are the only two possibilities. Scientific evidence suggests that these views are overly simplistic. In fact, there are many equivalent ways to shape the tongue for correct-sounding /r/, and they are distributed widely across the normal American English population.

Figures 5.1, 5.4a, and 5.4b illustrate the cross-speaker variability of /r/. Figures 5.4a and 5.4b show the differences in tongue shapes for /r/ first recorded in the 1960s by X-ray equipment of American English speakers producing running speech in an upright position. As noted above, Figure 5.1 shows midsagittal tongue configuration data for 12 American English speakers producing sustained /r/ while lying down. An even more varied set of MRIs can be found in Tiede (2004).

Because most traditional phoneticians have worked without access to modern imaging technology, awareness that American English speakers use more than one or two different tongue shapes for /r/, has spread very slowly. Before 1967, many phoneticians had observed that it was possible to produce /r/ using either the tongue tip or the tongue dorsum as the primary articulator, but their work was not widely cited. These two main types of /r/ were called "retroflex" and "bunched" (or "molar") /r/. Figure 5.4a shows the difference between the two types of tongue configuration. The tongue configuration for the "bunched" version is superimposed on the "retroflex" tongue configuration. The examples in Figure 5.4a came from an X-ray study whose results for /r/ are reported in Kent (1993) and in Shriberg and Kent (1982), among others. The discussion of

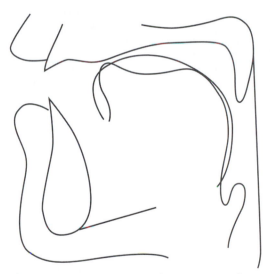

Figure 5.4a Superimposed (one on top of the other) examples of classic "bunched" and "retroflex" tongue configurations for /r/, based on X-ray tracings from same speaker. (Adapted from Kent, 1993.)

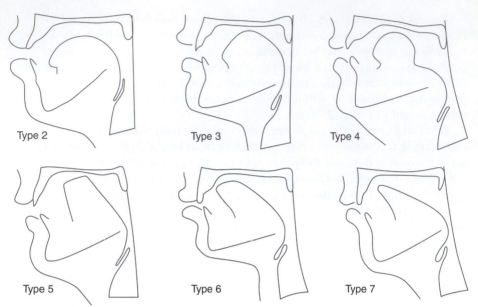

Figure 5.4b Types of American English tongue configurations for /r/ as identified by Delattre and Freeman (1968) from X-ray tracings of 44 subjects. Only Types 3 to 7 come from "rhotic" dialects. Type 3 is most like the description of the classic "bunched" type. Type 7 fits the description of the classic "retroflex" type. Types 4, 5, and 6 do not fit the classic descriptions. All types except Type 2 were found in both prevocalic and postvocalic positions. (Note that /r/ in postvocalic position is often written with /ɚ/ symbol.) Type 2 reflects the postvocalic schwa found in non-rhotic dialects (e.g. "fire" produced as "faa" /fɑː/, or "fayuh" /fajə/). Type 1 reflected a British /r/, and is not pictured here. (Figure adapted by Hagiwara (1995) from Delattre and Freeman (1968) and reprinted with permission.)

/r/ in Chapter 2 and in this chapter is organized according to this traditional definition of the two main types.

Delattre and Freeman (1968) changed the prevailing view somewhat when they took X-ray images of a large number of subjects producing /r/ in prevocalic and postvocalic or syllabic position. They sorted the American /r/'s they found into six categories, of which five occurred in rhotic dialects. Figure 5.4b shows these six types. Note that Type 2 produces the r-colored schwa, or schwar, of American English non-rhotic dialects. Types 3 to 7 produce "correct" /r/ as heard in American English rhotic dialects. Although some rhotic subjects switched tongue shapes, there were no clear overall patterns of change for /r/ according to pre- versus postvocalic position or regional version of rhotic dialect.

Although the 1968 Delattre and Freeman study was well known among phonetic scientists, it remained largely unknown and uncited among more applied users of phonetics knowledge (but cf. Shriberg and Kent, 1982; and Creaghead, Newman, and Secord, 1985, 1989). Thus, the majority of phonetics textbooks in current use among speech pathologists describe only one tongue configuration for /r/. For instance, Edwards (1997) and Parker (1982) describe only a "retro-flex" tongue position for /r/, while Morley (1979) describes only the "bunched" variety of /r/.

More recent X-ray, ultrasound, point-tracking, and MRI studies have con-firmed the multiplicity of tongue configurations for /r/ (Zawadazki and Kuehn, 1980; Alwan, Narayanan, et al., 1997; Ong and Stone 1998; Westbury et al., 1998; Guenther, Espy-Wilson, et al., 1999), although no consensus on classification has been reached. Figure 5.1 illustrates the variability in question.

Some obvious questions arise in the face of this demonstrated variability:

1. Do all of these configurations have the same IPA description?
2. Are particular tongue configurations characteristic of dialect?
3. Do all tongue configurations for /r/ sound the same?
4. How variable are "rhotic" sounds compared to other sounds?
5. What does variability mean for clinical work of teaching /r/?
6. How can such different tongue shapes produce such similar acoustics—that is, why do all these tongue shapes sound like /r/?

These questions are answered below, in order.

1. **How variable is rhotic /r/?** As Figure 5.1 shows, there are clearly several methods of configuring the vocal tract to produce an acceptable American English /r/. Other investigators support this point (Delattre and Freeman, 1968; Lindau, 1985; Wesbury et al., 1998; Hagiwara, 1995; Alwan et al., 1997; Espy-Wilson et al., 2000). There is no consensus at this time regarding how many different varieties exist. The Delattre and Freeman categorization is generally used as a guideline. Additional midsagittal MRIs of /r/ can be found in Alwan et al. (1997), and Tiede et al. (2004).

2. **Do all variants have the same IPA description?** Phonetics text-books deal with /r/ in several ways. Some phonetics textbooks refer to /r/ as made (i.e., having its primary constriction) at the alveolar place of articulation. The IPA symbol of an upside down /r/, or /ɹ/, which is often used for American English /r/ in the linguistics literature, can be used for a dental, alveolar or post-alveolar approximant (Handbook of the International Phonetic Association, 2005). In Chapter 2, this symbol is given as an alter-nate for "retroflex" /r/. Other textbooks refer to /r/ as having a post-alveolar place of articulation, while a third set describe it merely as palatal. But in fact, as Figure 5.1 shows, native speakers of American English produce /r/ with constrictions at several points along the palate, including the alveolar, post-alveolar, and mid-palatal places of articulation. For example, speakers 2, 5, 10, and 11 seem to make a narrow oral constriction with their tongue tips at the alveolar ridge. These /r/ variants would be described as voiced alveolar approximants. The rest of the speakers shown in Figure 5.1 seem to make their narrowest oral constriction at more posterior places along

the palate. These would be described in IPA terms as voiced post-alveolar or palatal approximants. It is worth noting that the slight backwards curl of the tongue that we call "retroflex," seen for speaker 5 of Figure 5.1, appears to be fairly uncommon among American English speakers.

Phonetic textbooks frequently do not discuss length of constriction for /r/ sounds. Retroflex /r/ types, where the constriction is alveolar, have shorter constrictions—that is, a smaller area of the tongue is brought closer to the palate. Bunched /r/ types, where the constriction is post-alveolar, have longer constrictions. The reason is that the tip of the tongue is particularly independent of the rest of the tongue. It is very difficult to raise the blade of the tongue to the palate without including some of the dorsum and the tongue tip. This effect can be seen in most of the "bunched" configurations in Figure 5.1. Note that long constrictions require two contiguous areas of the tongue to be activated in response to motor commands: e.g., a long palatal constriction involves precise positioning of both the tongue tip and blade, while a long post-alveolar constriction involves the tongue blade and dorsum. In other words, long constrictions require precise positioning of two or more points along the tongue. The ability to control more than one area of constriction along the tongue is a late-emerging skill in children.

The reason for the incomplete description of /r/ offered in phonetics books stems from the historical lack of imaging data, plus the fact that /r/ involves very little tactile feedback. In other words, without imaging data and tactile feedback, even phoneticians can guess wrongly about tongue shape.

3. **Do all tongue configurations sound the same?** A better way to phrase this question is: Do all configurations sound like "correct" American English /r/ to native ears? The answer is absolutely yes. Each speaker whose tongue configuration is shown in Figures 5.1, 5.4a, and 5.4b was a native speaker of (rhotic) American English with normal pronunciation of "correct" /r/. None of the speakers of Figure 5.1 show the r-colored schwa of Type 2 of Delattre and Freeman.

4. **Are different tongue configurations related to dialect region?** The short answer is that within the rhotic dialects, tongue configuration seems to follow no regional or social grouping. The evidence on hand from articulatory studies suggests that people from the same region show considerable variation in /r/ type. That is, the wide range of tongue shapes shown in Figure 5.1 might be seen in any group of native speakers from any part of North America. The crucial factor is that they be speakers of a rhotic dialect.

The long answer is that it would take a great deal of imaging data from hundreds of speakers across North America to answer the question definitively. Such a database of X-ray, ultrasound, and MRIs does not exist at present. It appears that that tongue configuration is characteristic of individuals rather than social groups. As noted above, however, the retroflex tongue shapes appear to be less common than other types across the normal population of American English speakers.

5. **Is this level of variability true for other sounds?** The answer is that /r/ seems to be an unusual case. The exact method of production varies for most sounds from individual to individual. For instance, speakers vary a good deal in the amount they round their lips for vowels such as /o/ and /u/, or consonants such as /s/ and /ʃ/. Similarly, speakers of American English vary a good deal in how much nasalization they produce during vowels. Some speakers raise their tongue tip to the alveolar ridge to produce "apical" /s/, while others use their tongue dorsum and angle the tongue tip down to produce "laminal" /s/ (Bladen and Nolan, 1977). Both methods produce a normal-sounding /s/. In addition, for the same tongue position, some speakers use the jaw muscles more than tongue muscles, while others barely move the jaw and use the tongue primarily.

However, the range of variability for other sounds is much less than that of /r/. Figure 5.5 illustrates this variability, by showing /l/ produced by the same speakers as in Figure 5.1. The figure shows that tongue shape variability in /l/ production is much less than in /r/ production. In addition, although tongue shapes for other sounds vary along a continuum, tongue shapes such as the classic "bunched" and "retroflex" /r/ are so different as to belong to different articulatory categories.

Lack of Acoustic Specificity for Tongue Shape

As noted above, and as shown in Figure 5.1, there are many articulatory types of /r/, and they all sound equally correct. Acoustically, /r/ sounds like /r/ as long as the third formant is very low. Hagiwara (1995) found that most normal-sounding speakers showed a third formant 30–40% below their average third formant for vowels. The minimum degree of lowering, for /r/ to sound like /r/, was 20%. The spectrogram panel of Figure 5.2a shows a vertical line drawn at the midpoint of /r/, where the third formant is lowest. Recent work on acoustic modeling of different /r/ shapes has shown that lowering F3 to such an extent requires the formation of a very large open space, or cavity, in the mouth. In most cases, this large cavity is in the front of the mouth, between the lip constriction and the palatal constriction (Alwan et al., 1997; Espy-Wilson et al., 2003; Zhang et al., 2005); but for speakers who use "retroflex" /r/, this cavity may be between the palatal and pharyngeal constrictions (Zhang et al., 2003). Note that although the tongue shapes in Figure 5.1 are very different, they all show a large cavity in the front of the mouth. Moving the palatal constriction backwards by moving the tongue back along the palate, raising the tongue tip so as to open up a space underneath, and protruding the lips all have the same effect of enlarging the front cavity. A client whose /r/ is not quite right may be able to improve it by using one of these articulatory strategies for increasing the size of the front cavity. In summary, the larger the front cavity, the lower the third formant, and the more /r/-like the sound.

It is worth pointing out that the greater the variability a listener has to contend with, the harder it is to learn how to position the vocal tract to reproduce that

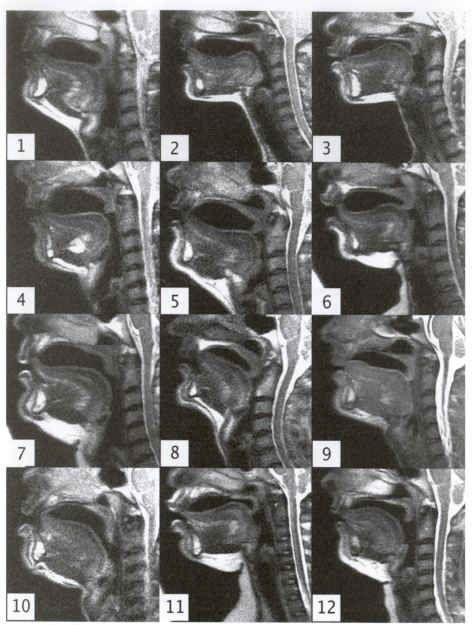

Figure 5.5 Midsagittal MRIs of speakers in Figure 5.1 producing sustained /l/. Similar vocal tract shapes have been recorded dynamically from prevocalic positions. (These images are reproduced from an ongoing research study sponsored by the U.S. National Institute of Deafness and Other Communication Disorders (R01 DC 005250, P.I. Suzanne Boyce).)

sound. The fact that speakers use so many different tongue shapes for /r/, with a similar acoustic spectrum, means that clues to pronunciation from listening are much more subtle, unreliable, and easily missed for /r/ than for any other sound.

The Science Behind the Techniques

What do all these facts about the articulation and acoustics of /r/ mean for teaching clients to produce the sound correctly? The simple answer is that *one size probably doesn't fit all*. The variability we see in tongue shape from normal speaker to normal speaker suggests that there are several different solutions to the problem of producing /r/. Since we know that no speaker's vocal tract is the same, it is likely that some solutions do not work for some vocal tracts. In other words, what works for one client (or clinician) may not work for another client. The clinician's task is to find a tongue configuration that works for the client. Therefore, a clinician must be *flexible in terms of the tongue configuration target*. If a clinician restricts therapy to a single definition of the tongue shape used to produce "correct" /r/, she may encounter considerable frustration if that tongue shape is not best suited to the client.

In fact, many techniques discussed in Chapter 2 for eliciting /r/ may be explained in part by the range of tongue configurations that can be used to produce it. In other words, some techniques are more suited to "shape" particular tongue configurations for /r/. These techniques then affect the shaping of the pharyngeal constriction for /r/, the length and placement of the constriction along the palate (alveolar or post-alveolar, short or long), and the degree of lip rounding.

The following section discusses the principles behind some of the techniques in Chapter 2, reasons why they work, and reasons why they may not work in particular cases. The chapter finishes with examples of how certain techniques can be associated with particular tongue shapes for "correct" /r/.

Pharyngeal Constriction

As mentioned earlier, the fact that /r/ involves a constriction in the pharynx comes as a surprise to most speech pathologists and phoneticians. This is because historically, the degree to which the tongue root moves for /r/ was not well known before the advent of MRI data. However, we know from acoustic studies that the pharyngeal constriction can be a crucial step in producing "correct" /r/ (Boyce et al., 1997; Espy-Wilson et al., 2000).

Several of the techniques listed in Chapter 2 are effective precisely because they start from a pharyngeal constriction and maintain it as the palatal constriction is added. A straightforward example is the process of shaping /r/ by starting with the vowel /ɑ/. While described simply as a "back" vowel in most phonetic textbooks, /ɑ/ is primarily made with a constriction in the pharynx between the tongue root and the pharyngeal wall. This pharyngeal aspect of /ɑ/ can be seen in Figure 5.6, which shows midsagittal MRIs of the vocal tract for the vowels /ɑ/, /i/, and /u/. As the figure shows, the massing of the tongue in the pharynx to produce a constriction has the effect of lowering the tongue dorsum, tip, and blade in the oral part of the vocal tract. (The feature designations [+low] and [+back] refer to the effect in the oral region.) Most of the tongue configurations for /r/ shown in Figure 5.1 also show pharyngeal constrictions.

Since /ɑ/ has a pharyngeal constriction, starting with this posture may encourage a tongue configuration for /r/ with a strong pharyngeal construction. From the vowel /ɑ/, there are two possible next steps in shaping /r/. One possibility is to coax the client to move the tongue dorsum up toward the palate while continuing to produce /ɑ/. The result should be a configuration similar to 3, 6, 7, or 12 in Figure 5.1. Another possibility is to coax the client to move the tongue tip up just behind the alveolar ridge. The result should be a configuration similar to 2, 5, 8, 9, or 11 in Figure 5.1. Depending on the exact dimensions of a client's vocal tract, any of these configurations may produce successful /r/.

The key point is that the client makes and maintains pharyngeal constriction while shaping /r/. However, because the tongue articulators are interconnected, the act of moving the tongue dorsum or tip upwards in the oral cavity may pull the tongue root away from the pharyngeal wall to some degree. This probably explains why the pharyngeal constrictions for /r/ shown in Figure 5.1 are generally wider than those shown for /ɑ/ in Figure 5.6.

It is not necessary to begin with /ɑ/ in order to achieve a pharyngeal constriction. For instance, some of the techniques mentioned in this chapter shape /r/ from /l/. As Figure 5.5 shows, some (but not all) speakers produce /l/'s with a bulge of the tongue dorsum and root in the pharynx. If the client is already able to produce a normal-sounding /l/, then he may already be making a constriction in the pharynx. If so, it is worth experimenting with shaping the /r/ sound by beginning with an /l/. Adding instructions to inhibit the /l/, as discussed in Chapter 2, may result in a configuration similar to that for 12 in Figure 5.1.

Some of the techniques discussed in Chapter 2 shape /r/ by starting from something close to its palatal constriction. For instance, it may seem intuitively

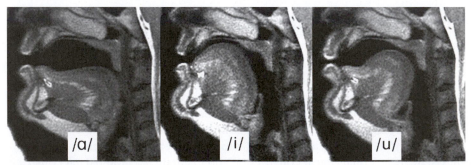

Figure 5.6 Midsagittal MRIs of three sustained vowels spoken by a male speaker of an American English rhotic dialect (7 of Figure 5.1). The vowels are /ɑ/ as in "cot," /i/ as in "see," and /u/ as in "moon." (Images reproduced from an ongoing research study sponsored by the U.S. National Institute of Deafness and Other Communication Disorders (R01 DC 005250, P.I. Suzanne Boyce).)

obvious that "retroflex" /r/, which has a constriction in the alveolar/post-alveolar location along the palate, can be shaped from /i/, which also has a post-alveolar constriction (see Figure 5.6). The /r/ configurations shown in 5, 8, 9, and 11 in Figure 5.1 fit this description. However, the /i/ sound is typically made with a very wide pharynx, because the effort of moving the tongue tip and blade as far forward as the alveolar ridge typically pulls the rest of the tongue forward as well. (Note that this posture of a wide pharynx is why we typically tell clients to produce /i/ when we want to visualize the larynx from above, as in flexible endoscopy.) However, as Figure 5.1 shows, all types of /r/ are made with the pharynx narrower than for /i/, and some /r/ configurations have a very narrow pharyngeal constriction. If /r/ is shaped from /i/, the client may imitate the pharyngeal width of /i/ as well as the location of the tongue tip/blade constriction. If so, guide the client to narrow the pharynx in some way. Sometimes, merely telling the client to tighten tongue muscles in the pharynx is enough to produce the /r/ quality.

Vowel "Substitutes" for /r/

"Incorrect" /r/ may sound like any vowel, but it most frequently sounds like a schwa vowel, written in phonetic font as /ə/ or /ʌ/. (This is often referred to as the substitution of schwa for /r/.) It sounds like schwa rather than some other vowel because the tongue root placement (i.e., the pharyngeal constriction) is similar to that for a central vowel (Gick et al., 2002). Thus, if incorrect /r/ sounds like schwa, the clinician knows that the client has produced appropriate movement of the tongue root toward pharyngeal constriction. At the same time, the lack of sufficient /r/-coloring is a clue that movement of the tip/blade or blade/ dorsum (for any type of /r/) toward the palate, to form a front cavity, is insufficient in some way. In other words, the substitution of schwa for /r/ reflects the fact that only one of the two required tongue constrictions for /r/ (the pharyngeal constriction) has occurred at the time.

The missing palatal constriction has two possible causes. First, the movement of the tongue toward the palatal constriction for /r/ may be timed correctly but may not be strong enough to form a consonant-sized narrow gap between palate and tongue. In such a case, teach the client to decrease the gap between the palate and the tongue to increase the degree of /r/ coloring until he can produce a correct /r/. A second potential cause is incorrect timing: the client may be using postvocalic /r/ timing (in which the palatal constriction follows the pharyngeal constriction) and the movement of the tongue toward the palate may occur too late. The result sounds like a schwa vowel. In this case, use techniques to change the timing of the pharyngeal constriction movement versus the palatal constriction movement.

Sides of the Tongue

A third possible cause of vowel sound for /r/ comes from the fact the sides of the tongue are less crucial for vowels. As with /l/, both the sides and the tip of the tongue must work together. For /r/'s where the tongue tip is raised, as in 2,

5, 6, 8, 9, 10, 11, and 12 in Figure 5.1, the sides of the tongue are raised (rather than lowered, as for /l/). For many of these /r/'s, the tongue sides make contact with the upper teeth in the far back of the palate. These /r/ configurations can be "shaped" from /l/ by changing the orientation of the tongue sides. The classically "bunched" /r/'s seen in 1, 3, 4, and 7 in Figure 5.1 pull the sides of the tongue in toward the middle; the tongue loses its flatness and becomes more mounded. A similar mounded configuration of the tongue sides is characteristic of /u/. Thus, moving from an /i/ configuration or an /l/ configuration to an /u/ configuration may help the client pull his sides of the tongue into the middle to produce a "bunched" /r/. If a "correct" /r/ is not achieved with this maneuver by itself, then have the client tighten the pharynx temporarily. Several techniques described in Chapter 2 are effective because they follow this theory.

Relevance to Clinical Practice

The next section connects the science of /r/ to clinical practice. The elicitation techniques for /r/ and /ɚ/ in Chapter 2 are presented again below. They are listed again to direct the clinician to the specific tongue shapes that each technique can elicit, based on Figure 5.1, 1 through 12. In some instances additional points of clarification are provided when necessary. Techniques marked with a ★ are good starting points for therapy, since they have the potential to elicit a wide range of different /r/ and /ɚ/ types. This integration of science and practice should help clinicians achieve new levels of success in eliciting /r/ sounds.

Prevocalic /r/

Eliciting Techniques

1. Show the client how to raise his tongue (i.e., curl the tongue upward or point the tongue downward in retroflexed and bunched postures, respectively). Use a tongue depressor to guide the movement if necessary. Hold the lips still to focus attention on the tongue movement.

   In Figure 5.1, 5 and 7 can be used for illustration to a client. The directions for raising the tongue tip may result in any tongue shape with tongue tip up. Images with the tongue tip up are 2, 5, 6, 8, 9, 10, 11, or 12.

   The directions for pointing the tongue tip down may result in any tongue shape with the tip down.

   Images with tongue tip down are 1, 5, and 7.

2. Illustrations of tongue placement are helpful for some individuals. Try illustrating tongue position with hand gestures. Hold one hand horizontally to represent the tongue. With your other hand underneath, demonstrate the tongue movement for /r/ (e.g., "bunched" posture). Have the client cup his

hand to indicate that the tongue tip is raised and slightly curled back (e.g., "retroflexed" posture).

See 5 and 7 in Figure 5.1.

3. Tell the client to place his tongue tip behind his upper front teeth. Use a tongue depressor to assist the client in positioning the tongue by asking him to place the lingual tip on the "shelf." Next, instruct the client to curl the tongue backward without touching the roof of the mouth until it cannot go back any farther. Finally, tell the client to lower the jaw slightly and attempt to produce /ru/ (e.g., "retroflexed" posture).

See 5 in Figure 5.1.

★4. To establish the retroflex /r/, Bauman-Waengler (2004) recommends a "sweeping" action using the following steps:

   a. Show the client how to raise the tongue behind the alveolar ridge without making contact with this articulator.
   b. Have the client raise the posterior edges of the tongue to touch the upper molars.
   c. Introduce movement by having the client "sweep" the palatal area. Instruct him to glide the tongue while touching the alveolar area, backward and forward, while "sweeping" the palatal area.
   d. Next have the client open his mouth slightly and repeat the sweeping movement without touching the tip of the tongue or palatal area while keeping the edges of the tongue raised, and then adding voicing. As the tongue edges are raised and voicing is added, the client should produce an r-like sound.

See 2, 5, 6, 8, 9, 10, 11, and 12 in Figure 5.1.

★5. Direct the client to stick out his tongue. Using a tongue depressor, touch the edges of the tongue. Then use the depressor to touch the gum areas along side the upper molars. Next, tell the client to bring the tongue back into the mouth while raising the tongue to make the edges of his tongue contact the upper teeth where you just touched (e.g., the "bunched" posture).

See 1, 3, 4, 6, 7, and 12 in Figure 5.1.

6. To inhibit /w/:

   a. Retract the lips slightly. Suggest trying a "small smile," or say "let the lips go to sleep," or "no kissing frogs."
   b. Place the client's forefinger crosswise on his lower lip. Tell him to concentrate on his tongue and move the whole body of the tongue forward.
   c. Position the mouth in a more open position at a distance that will not interfere with the tongue elevation.

See 1, 4, and 7 in Figure 5.1.

7. To inhibit the /j/, where the tongue is convex (Bauman-Waengler, 2004):
   a. Position the mouth in a more open posture.
   b. Roll the tongue so to achieve a medial lingual groove.

   See 1, 3, 4, and 7 in Figure 5.1.

★8. To inhibit the /l/:
   a. Release the tongue tip from the alveolar ridge.
   b. Raise the edges for the tongue to prevent lateral airflow.
   c. Move the tongue slightly backward.

   See any of the images in Figure 5.1.

★9. Remind the client to use the growling dog sound (grrr), the tiger sound (grrr), the growling sound, the race-car sound (ruh), the middle sound, the flowing sound, or the lifter sound (Lindamood and Lindamood, 1998).

   See any of the images in Figure 5.1.

Moto-Kinesthetic

★Using latex gloves, the clinician places the thumb and forefinger of one hand on the upper lip about an inch apart. The thumb and forefinger of the other hand are placed similarly on the lower lip. The mouth is open slightly to make the tongue visible. The lips are held firmly to inhibit rounding. When the /r/ is attempted, the lower jaw is moved downward toward the next vowel (Young and Hawk, 1955).

Refer to any of the images in Figure 5.1.

Sound Approximation

1. Shape /r/ from /ɚ/. Practice syllables that begin with /ɚ/ (e.g., /ɚrɑ, ɚri, ɚro/). *Warning*: Beware of the risk of ending up with /ɚ/ preceding all consonant /r/ words. If you use this exercise, teach the client to whisper /ɚ/ before the consonant /r/.

   See any of the images in Figure 5.1. This technique encourages a change from the postvocalic timing pattern of tongue root/dorsum movement before tongue tip/blade movement to the prevocalic timing pattern of simultaneous tongue root/dorsum and tongue tip/blade movement. Both timing patterns end in one of the appropriate tongue shapes for /ɚ/.

2. Separate /r/ from intervocalic /ɚr/ contexts that occur in certain words. The intervocalic /ɚr/ contains both the vocalic and consonant /r/. Individuals who can say or who have been taught the vowel first but say w/r often produce /r/ correctly in intervocalic contexts. Use these contexts to begin training (Slipakoff, 1967).

For example:

carry ⇒ care re ⇒ care read ⇒ read
caring ⇒ care ring ⇒ ring

3. For children, Garbutt and Anderson (1980) suggest distinguishing between two kinds of "R's," the standing R and the running R. They can be located in words containing the intervocalic /ɚr/ as in *marry*, *carry*, and *carrot*. The standing R "purrs" as in *her*. The running R as in *run* begins with the standing R. It needs the standing ɾ to make it run.

   See any of the images in Figure 5.1. This technique encourages a change from the postvocalic timing pattern of tongue root/dorsum movement before tongue tip/blade movement, to the prevocalic timing pattern of simultaneous tongue root/dorsum and tongue tip/blade movement. Both timing patterns end in one of the appropriate tongue shapes for /r/ (see Figure 5.3). Note also that the impression of /w/ occurs because the tongue root/dorsum position (i.e., pharyngeal constriction) occurs at the same time as lip constriction, producing a rounded back vowel sound.

4. Shape /r/ from /ʒ/. Instruct him to prolong /ʒ/ and then stop while holding that tongue position, then to think a silent /ɚ/ or /ʌ/ and say /rʌ/.

   This technique encourages a change from the postvocalic timing pattern of tongue root/dorsum movement before tongue tip/blade movement to the prevocalic timing pattern of simultaneous tongue root/dorsum and tongue tip/blade movement. Both timing patterns end in one of the appropriate tongue shapes for /r/.

5. Have the client practice the sequence /tʌ-dʌ-lʌ-rʌ/.

6. Shape /r/ from /t/ or /d/. Practice sequences /tʌ rʌ/→/tər/→/tr/. Instruct the client to pull his tongue back slightly while pointing the tongue tip in the direction of the pre-palatal area; then and lift the edges of the tongue to touch the back upper back teeth and say /r/ with emphasis.

   See 2, 5, 6, 8, 9, 10, and 12 of Figure 5.1. All preserve the instructions to point the tongue tip in the direction of the pre-palatal area. However, many speakers instinctively lower the tongue tip in anticipation of the vowel /ʌ/. A client who lowers the tip may produce an /r/ similar to 1, 4, or 7.

7. Shape /r/ from /n/. Practice: a) *none* (tongue back) *run* and b) /nʌ rə/ or /nə/-*run*.

   See the same images in Figure 5.1 as for /t/ or /d/ above.

8. Insert a silent /ɚ/ between /t/ and /r/, and /d/ and /r/ blends. Instruct the client to say *train*, *tree* or *dream*, *dry* and to insert a silent or whispered /ɚ/ after the initial consonant.

   See any of the images in Figure 5.1.

Additional Note

None of these techniques makes overt reference to the pharyngeal constriction. Sometimes a client will naturally make a pharyngeal constriction in response to the direction to pull the tongue back; but sometimes the client will struggle to maintain the pharyngeal constriction of the starting point sound. You may need to combine these techniques with other techniques that target the pharyngeal constriction. Two starting point sounds that include a pharyngeal constriction are /ɑ/ and /l/ (see *Figure 5.6 for /ɑ/ and Figure 5.5 for /l/*). If using these sounds as starting points, encourage the client to maintain the pharyngeal constriction while moving other areas of the tongue or vocal tract.

Postvocalic /ɚ/

Eliciting Techniques

1. Shriberg (1975) suggests seven articulatory requisites for /ɚ/:

   - Be able to move the body of the tongue grossly on command.
   - Know (by pointing with his finger) where his tongue tip is.
   - Know (by pointing) where his alveolar ridge is.
   - Be able to lift his tongue tip to his alveolar ridge.
   - Be able to sustain elevation of his tongue tip for at least five seconds without the tongue tip roving around.
   - Be able to move tongue body and tip forward and backward without jaw motion.
   - Be able to move and tense his tongue independently of phonation jaw movement.

★2. Instruct the client to growl like a tiger while you model the /ɚ/ to make a sound like a motor starting up.

   See all images of /ɚ/ presented in Figure 5.1.

★3. Have the client lie his back on a floor mat, relax the mouth, and say /ɚ/.

   See all images of /ɚ/ in Figure 5.1, but this technique is most relevant to 7 and 12.

4. Direct the client to lower the tongue tip and the draw the back of the tongue posteriorly, as for producing a silent /g/. Then tell the client to make the edges of the tongue touch the insides of the back teeth. Remind the client to turn on the voice box while producing /ɚ/.

   See 1, 3, 4, and 7 in Figure 5.1.

★5. Tell the client to open his mouth and make a silent /k/, and then to attempt the growling sound /ɚ/.

See 1, 3, 4, 7, 9, and 11 in Figure 5.1.

★6. Tell the client to open his mouth and to raise the tongue. Model the tongue tip in the center of the mouth almost touching the hard palate. Use a mirror if necessary. Then direct the client to close his mouth until his teeth are almost clenched and say /ɚ/ (e.g., "retroflexed" posture).

See 2, 5, 6, 8, 9, 10, and 12 in Figure 5.1.

7. Tell the client that you are going to pull on an imaginary string attached to the back of his head. As you pull the imaginary string up from the back of the client's head, instruct the client to lift the back of a tensed tongue and say /ɚ/. For the younger client, you may want to introduce this task by asking him to pretend he is a puppet (e.g., "bunched" posture).

See 1, 4, and 6 in Figure 5.1.

8. Show the client the shape of the lips and the height of the tongue in the production of /ɚ/. Have him feel the vibration on in his throat approximately where you would stimulate /k/. Although many clinicians focus on retracting the tongue tip, we believe you should show the height of the back of the tongue. Demonstrate by placing the tip of your tongue down behind your lower teeth and saying /ɚ/ to show the elevation of the back of the tongue (e.g., "bunched" posture). An alternative is to show the articulatory posture with the retraction of the tongue tip (e.g., "retroflexed" posture).

See 1 and 4 in Figure 5.1.

9. Use a tongue depressor to help the client attain the /ɚ/ posture. Slowly move the tongue back while the client is attempting to produce /ɚ/. Place the tip of a tongue depressor on the gum ridge behind the lower central incisors and ask the client to hold it there with the underside of the tongue. Move the tongue back with a lever action of the tongue depressor while the client is attempting /ɚ/.

See 1, 4, and 7 in Figure 5.1.

10. Show the curling movement of the tongue. Hold one hand out (palm down) to represent the tongue, and place the other hand underneath to represent the floor of the mouth. Move the upper hand to illustrate the backward curling action. You can also hold your hand out (palm up) and gradually curl your fingers upward. Have the client try this while attempting to produce /ɚ/. Some clients produce excessive lip rounding. To minimize the lip rounding, place your gloved thumb and forefingers at the corners of the client's lower lip, or lay a tongue depressor crosswise on his lower lip.

See 5, 9, and 11 in Figure 5.1.

11. Sometimes simply telling a client to place his tongue tip on the roof of his mouth and then to drop it off slightly while saying /ɚ/ works quite well.

Note: Be careful when you emphasize one gesture over another, since the client might adopt an exaggerated version of the sound.

See 5, 9, and 11 in Figure 5.1.

★12. Remind the client to use the growling dog sound (grrr), the tiger sound (grrr), the growling sound, the arm-wresting sound (errr), the middle sound, the flowing sound, or the lifter sound (Lindamood and Lindamood, 1998).

See all types of /ɚ/ in Figure 5.1.

Sound Approximation

★1. Shape /ɚ/ from the client's incorrect production. Instruct the client to sustain his error sound, and then provide cues for him to reposition the tongue. For example: "Lift your tongue—pull it back a little more—good, hold it— did you hear that?"

See all types of /ɚ/ in Figure 5.1.

2. Shape /ɚ/from /u/. Ask the client to say the middle sound in "put." Then tell him to prolong that sound. Next instruct him to slowly move his tongue backward. Use a tongue depressor to guide the movement if necessary. When the client produces /ɚ/, have him listen to the new sound. Then, have him stop saying the sound but hold the same tongue position while saying /ɚ/, without using that other /u/ sound. Sometimes you will need to tell the client to "turn that new sound on and off" before he can say /ɚ/ spontaneously.

See 1, 4, and 7 in Figure 5.1. These instructions affect the pharyngeal constriction the most.

3. Shape /ɚ/ from /ɑ/. Instruct the client to prolong /ɑ/, then slowly raise the tip of the tongue up and back. When /aɚ/ is attained, ask him to hold onto the end sound, which is /ɚ/. Use a tongue depressor to guide the movement of the tongue if necessary.

See 6 and 12 in Figure 5.1.

★4. Shape /ɚ/ from /ɛ/. Ask the client to say the word "bet," then prolong the vowel /ɛ/ in "bet." Then, slowly raise the tongue tip up and back to elicit /ɛɚ/. Instruct him to sustain the end of /ɛɚ/, which is /ɚ/. Guide movement with tongue depressor if necessary.

See 2, 5, 8, 9, 10, 11, and 12 in Figure 5.1.

5. Shape /ɚ/ from /i/. Have the client prolong the /i/ and simultaneously raise the tongue tip or pull the tongue back while keeping the sides of the tongue against the upper teeth.

If the tongue tip is raised, then see 6, 9, and 11 in Figure 5.1. If the tongue is moved back so that sides of the tongue touch the upper teeth, and the tongue tip remains low, then see 1, 3, 4, and 7.

★6. Shape /ɚ/ from /r/. Instruct the client to sustain the beginning part of the first sound of the word "run," then hold that sound like a purr.

See all images of /ɚ/ in Figure 5.1.

7. Shape /ɚ/ from /i/. Instruct him to prolong a tense /i/. While the client is saying the /i/, direct him to lift the tongue and curl back the tongue tip to say /ɚ/. An alternate is to ask the client to relax the lips and move the tongue back gradually to produce the /ɚ/.

If the tongue tip is raised, then see 6, 9, and 11 in Figure 5.1. If the tongue is moved back so that sides of the tongue touch the upper teeth, and the tongue tip remains low, then see 1, 3, 4, and 7 in Figure 5.1.

★8. Shape the /ɚ/ from /l/. Tell the client to sustain the /l/ sound while dragging the tip of the tongue slowly back along the roof of the mouth, so far back that you may need to drop the tongue tip slightly. Accompany the directions with hand gestures by moving the fingertips back slowly with the palm turned upward. You can also try this exercise while systematically increasing the rate of sequences of /lɚ-lɚ-lɚ/.

See 2, 5, 6, 8, 9, 10, 11, and 12 of Figure 5.1, depending on initial tongue shape for /l/.

9. Shape /ɚ/ from /d/. Instruct the client to raise his tongue and say /d/, then drop the tip of the tongue slightly and say /ɚ/.

See 2 and 10 in Figure 5.1.

10. Shape /ɚ/ from /z/. Tell the client to prolong the /z/ sound, lower the jaw, and pull the tongue back. Also, tell the client to say a hard or quick /z/ with tongue movement backward.

See 5, 9, 11, and 12 in Figure 5.1.

11. Shape /ɚ/ from /ʒ/. Ask the client to hold his tongue in the position for /ʒ/ while you lower his jaw.

This technique is best illustrated by reference to the voiceless cognate of /ʒ/. Because the jaw operates on a hinge, lowering the jaw from this vocal tract shape will pull the tip/blade of the tongue further down from the palate than the tongue dorsum. This will move the location of the constriction back, while also increasing the width of the constriction. The final vocal tract shape should resemble that of 1 or 3 in Figure 5.1.

12. Shape /ɚ/ from /n/. Instruct the client to spread the sides of his mouth with his fingers and prolong /n/. Then ask him to curl the tip of his tongue backward. As an alternative, instruct the client to make a really long /n/ (sustained /n/) while curling the tip of the tongue toward the roof of the mouth to produce the /ɚ/.

See 5 in Figure 5.1.

13. Shape /ɚ/ from /θ/ or /ð/. Instruct him to prolong /ð/ and pull the tip of the tongue back quickly and upward toward the alveolar ridge.

    See 2, 5, 6, 8, 9, 10, 11, and 12 in Figure 5.1.

14. Shape /ɚ/ from a /t/ and /d/. Practice the sequence /tɚ-dɚ-tɚ-dɚ/. Tell the client to pull his tongue back from /t/ and /d/.

    See all images of /ɚ/ in Figure 5.1, since the orientation of the tongue tip is not specified.

15. Ask children to imitate the purr of a kitten, a growl, or the crow of the rooster.

    See all images of /ɚ/ in Figure 5.1.

Summary

This chapter has reviewed the current state of knowledge on the articulation and acoustics of American English /r/, together with the clinical applications of that knowledge. In particular, the chapter set out to show the multiplicity of ways in which American English speakers produce /r/. The complicated nature of /r/ has always forced clinicians to "custom design" their strategies in therapy, but this has been largely a process of trial and error. As has become clear in recent years, much of the traditional knowledge taught to clinicians in phonetics courses about /r/ phonetics has been incomplete and in some cases misleading. This mismatch between traditional knowledge and clinical practice has been a source of frustration. Further, the ability of clinicians to use their knowledge of the fundamental science of phonetics to improve the practice of therapy has been reduced. Due to recent vocal tract imaging and tracking techniques, new information about phonetics and about /r/ in particular has become available. The goal of this chapter is to improve clinical understanding of the fundamental factors involved in correct /r/ production, which should result in improved practice, happier clinicians, and happier clients.

The main points of the chapter are summarized here:

1. American English speakers produce /r/ with a multiplicity of tongue shapes. These are illustrated in Figure 5.1 and Figures 5.4a and 4b.

2. For speakers of rhotic dialects, prosodic variables, such as stress or word position, do not by themselves cause systematic change in overall tongue shape, such as a switch from retroflex to bunched /r/. In other words, the older phonetic tradition of using different symbols for stressed and unstressed /r/, or consonantal versus syllabic /r/, should not be understood to imply that these sounds involve significantly different tongue shapes. There may well be systematic differences in tongue shape for non-rhotic dialects.

3. The timing of tongue tip/blade toward constriction at the palate and of tongue dorsum/root movement toward constriction at the pharynx is different for prevocalic and postvocalic /r/. This is relatively new information, and it explains why some clinical techniques are more effective with prevocalic or with postvocalic /r/. Teaching a client to produce both effectively means teaching two patterns of timing.

4. Most speakers of American English rhotic dialects do not change tongue shapes in different phonetic contexts. However, some speakers do appear to switch under some circumstances. Guenther et al. (1999) found that speakers who use a "retroflex" tongue shape (similar to 5 in Figure 5.1) in all other contexts tend to use a "bunched" shape in a /gr/ cluster. Tiede et al. (2005) found that some speakers switch tongue shapes in different /i/, /u/, and /ɑ/ vowel contexts. (The "bunched" and "retroflex" tongue shapes shown in Figure 5.4a come from different phonetic contexts.) The factors that lead a speaker to switch tongue shapes are not well understood at this time. However, if a client has more trouble with /r/ in particular phonetic contexts, use a teaching technique aimed at eliciting a different tongue shape.

5. In order for an /r/ to sound like a correct /r/, the acoustic profile must include a very low third formant (F3). The client must make a very large, open, front cavity between the lips and the palatal constriction. Moving the palatal constriction back, raising the tongue tip, and protruding the lips all have the effect of increasing the size of the front cavity and thus lowering F3. Experimenting with the size of the front cavity can be particularly helpful when the client's /r/ is close but not ideally /r/-like.

6. The pharyngeal constriction is very important to the correct production of /r/. Further, speakers have limited intuition about the shape of their pharynx, including the presence or absence of a pharyngeal constriction. When told to move the back of the tongue, for instance, some clients may move the tongue root, while others may move only the tongue blade or dorsum. Techniques that shape /r/ from sounds with a pharyngeal constriction, such as /l/ and /i/, may encourage correct pharyngeal constriction. They may also encourage postvocalic /r/ timing, where pharyngeal constriction must precede palatal constriction.

7. The multiplicity of tongue shapes used by different speakers probably means that what works for one vocal tract may not work well for another. Examples of factors that influence what works include palate shape, which affects the space available for the front cavity, pharyngeal length and width, and tongue size. Many adults and particularly children are not skillful at controlling constriction at multiple points along the tongue, together with the orientation of tongue sides. Thus, clinicians should experiment with different tongue shapes and different techniques. For example, "retroflex" tongue shapes have raised tongue sides from the tip to the root, while more "bunched" shapes are flat near the palatal constriction and have raised sides in the tongue root area.

Most of the points listed above are based on new information about the fundamental acoustic and articulatory science of /r/ and /ɚ/. This chapter is based on the premise that this new knowledge will help clinicians understand how and why the techniques in this book are successful.

References

Alwan, A., Narayanan, S., & Haker, K. (1997). Towards articulatory-acoustic models of liquid consonants Part II: The Rhotics." *Journal of the Acoustical Society of America, 101*(2), 1078–1089.

Bauman-Waengler, J. (2004). *Articulatory and Phonological Impairments.* Boston, MA: Allyn and Bacon, Inc.

Bernthal, J., & Bankson, N. (1981). *Articulation disorders.* Englewood Cliffs, NJ: Prentice-Hall.

Bernthal, J.A., & Bankson, N.W. (2004). *Articulation and Phonological Disorders.* Boston, MA: Allyn and Bacon, Inc.

Bleile, K.M. (1996). *Articulation and Phonology Disorders: A Book of Exercises.* San Diego, CA: Singular Publishing Group, Inc.

Bleile, K.M. (2004). *Manual of Articulation and Phonological Disorders Infancy through Adulthood.* Clifton Park, NY: Delmar Learning.

Boyce, S., & Espy-Wilson, C. (1997). Coarticulatory stability in American English /r/. *Journal of the Acoustical. Society of America, 101,* 3741–3753.

Browman, C., & Goldstein, L. (1992). Articulatory Phonology: An Overview. *Phonetica, 9,* 155–180.

Celce-Murcia, M., Brinton, D., & Goodwin, J. (1997). *Teaching Pronunciation: A Reference for Teachers of English to Speakers of Other Languages.* Cambridge, UK: Cambridge University Press.

Catford, J.C. (1988). *A Practical Introduction to Phonetics.* Oxford: Clarendon Press.

Creaghead, N.A., Newman, P.W., & Secord, W.A. (1989). *Assessment and Remediation of Articulatory and Phonological Disorders.* Columbus, OH: Merrill Publishing Company, 1989.

Dale, P., & Poms, L. (1994). *English Pronunciation for International Students.* Englewoood Cliffs, NJ: Prentice Hall Regents, 1994.

Delattre, P., & Freeman, D. (1968). A dialect study of American r's by X-ray Motion Picture. *Linguistics, 44,* 29–68.

Espy-Wilson, C., Boyce, S., Jackson, M., Narayanan, S., & Alwan, A. (2000). Acoustic Modeling of American English /r/. *Journal of the Acoustical Society of America, 108*(1), 343–356.

Garbutt, C., & Anderson, J. (1980). *Effective methods for correcting articulatory defects.* Danville, IL.: Interstate.

Gick, B., Campbell, F., Oh, S., & Tamburri-Watt, L. (2006). Toward universals in the gestural organization of syllables: A cross-linguistics study of liquids. *Journal of Phonetics, 34,* 49–72.

Gick, B., Kang, M., & Whalen, D. (2002). MRI evidence for commonality in the post-oral articulations of English vowels and liquids, *Journal of Phonetics, 30*(3), 357–371.

Gordon-Brannan, M.E., & Weiss, C.E. (2007). *Clinical Management of Articulatory and Phonologic Disorders.* (3rd Edition). Baltimore, MD: Lippincott Williams & Wilkins.

Hagiwara, R. (1995). Acoustic realizations of American /r/ as produced by women and men. *UCLA Phonetics Laboratory Working Papers, 90,* 1–187.

Flowers, A.M. (1980). *The big book of sounds.* Danville, IL: The Interstate Printers and Publishers, Inc.

Kent, R. (1988). Normal aspects of articulation. In Bernthal & Bankson (Eds.), *Articulation and phonological disorders.* (4th Edition). Boston, MA: Allyn & Bacon.

Klein, E. S. (1996). *Clinical phonology assessment and treatment of articulation disorders in children and adults.* San Diego, CA: Singular Publishing Group, Inc.

Krakow, R. (1999). Physiological organization of syllables: A review. *Journal of Phonetics, 27,* 23–54.

Ladefoged, P. (2001). *A course in phonetics.* (4th Edition). Fort Worth, TX: Harcourt Brace.

Labov, William W., Ash, S., & Boberg, C. (2005). *The atlas of North American English.* New York: Mouton de Gruyter.

Lindamood, P., & Lindamood, P. (1998). *The Lindamood Phoneme Sequencing Program for Reading, Spelling, and Speech.* Austin, TX: Pro-Ed.

Lindau, M. (1985). The story of /r/. In Fromkin, V. (Ed.), *Phonetic Linguistics: Essays in Honor of Peter Ladefoged*, 157–168. Orlando, FL: Academic Press.

Pena-Brooks, A., & Hedge, M.N. (2000). *Assessment and treatment of articulations and phonological disorders of children*. Austin, TX: Pro-Ed.

McDonald, E. (1964). *Articulation testing and treatment: A sensory motor approach.* Pittsburgh, PA: Stanwix.

Ristuccia, C., & Shine, R. (2004). Got /R/ problems? A context-specific phonetic treatment methodology for /R/. *Annual Convention of the American Speech-Language-Hearing Association,* Philadelphia, PA. Retrievable from the World Wide Web: http://www.sayitright.com.

Roth, F.P., & Worthington, C.K. (2001). *Treatment resource manual for speech-language pathology*. Clifton Park, NY: Thomson Delmar Learning.

Scripture, M., & Jackson, E. (1927). *A manual of exercises for the correction of speech disorders.* Philadelphia, PA: F.A. Davis.

Secord, W., & Shine, R. (2003). *S-CAT: Secord Contextual Articulation Tests.* Greenville, SC: Super Duper Publications, Inc.

Secord, W., & Donohue, J. (2002). *CAAP: Clinical Assessment of Articulation and Phonology.* Greenville, SC: Super Duper Publications, Inc.

Shriberg, L., & Kent, R. (1982). Clinical phonetics. New York, NY: Macmillan.

Shriberg, L. (1975). A response program for evoking /E/. *Journal of Speech and Hearing Disorders, 40,* 92–105.

Slipakoff, E. (1967). An approach to correction of defective /r/. *Journal of Speech and Hearing Disorders, 32,* 71–75.

Small, L. (2005). *Fundamentals of phonetics: A practical guide for students*. Boston, MA: Pearson.

Smit, A.B. (2004). *Articulation and phonology resource guide for school-age children and adults.* Clifton Park, NY: Thomson Delmar Learning.

Sproat, R., & Fujimura, O. (1993). Allophonic variation in English /l/ and its implications for phonetic implementation. *Journal of Phonetics, 21,* 291–311.

Stevens, K., & Keyser, S. (1989). Primary features and their enhancement in consonants. *Language, 65,* 81–106.

Stone, M. (1995). How the tongue takes advantage of the palate during speech. In Bell-Berti, F., & Raphael, L. (Eds.), *Producing speech: Contemporary issues for Katherine Safford Harris,* 143–154. New York, NY: AIP Press.

Van Riper. C. (1963). *Speech correction: Principles and methods.* Englewood Cliffs, NJ: Prentice-Hall.

Van Riper, C. (1978). *Speech correction: Principles and methods.* (6th Edition). Englewood Cliffs, NJ: Prentice-Hall.

Van Riper, C., & Emerick, L. (1984). *Speech correction: Principles and methods.* Englewood Cliffs, NJ: Prentice-Hall.

Weiss, C., Lillywhite, H., & Gordon, M. (1987). *Clinical management of articulation disorders. (*2nd Edition*).* St. Louis: C.V. Mosby.

Westbury, J. R., Hashi, M., and Lindstrom, M. J. (1999). Differences among speakers in lingual articulation of American English /r/. *Speech Communication, 26,* 203–226.

Young, E., & Hawk, S. (1955). *Moto-kinesthetic speech training.* Stanford, CA: Stanford University Press.

Zawadzki, P., & Kuehn, D. (1980). A cineradiographic study of statis and dynamic aspects of American English /r/. *Phonetica, 37,* 253–266.

Other Resources

Berry, M., & Eisenson, J. (1956). *Speech disorders: Principles and practices of therapy.* New York: Appleton-Century-Crofts.

Eisenson, J., & Ogilvie, M. (1957). *Speech correction in the schools.* New York: Macmillan.

Fisher, H. (1975). *Improving voice and articulation.* Boston, MA: Houghton Mifflin.

Haycock, G. (1964). *The teaching of speech.* Washington, DC: The Volta Bureau.

Johnson, J. (1980). *Nature and treatment of articulation disorders.* Springfield, IL: Charles C. Thomas.

Irwin, R. (1965). *Speech and hearing therapy.* Pittsburgh, PA: Stanwix-House.

Ling, D. (1976). *Speech and the hearing impaired child: Theory and practice.* Washington, DC: The Alexander Graham Bell Association for the Deaf.

Milisen, R.A. (1954). A rationale for articulation disorders. *Journal of Speech and Hearing Disorders,* Monograph Supplement 4, 5–18.

Nemoy, E., & Davis, S. (1954). *The correction of defective consonant sounds.* Magnolia, MA: Expression Co.

Parker, J. (1975). *My speech workbook.* (Book 1). Danville, IL: Interstate.

Parker J. (1976). *My speech workbook.* (Book 2). Danville, IL: Interstate.

Parker, J. (1978). *My speech workbook.* (Book 3). Danville, IL: Interstate.

Parker, J. (1980). *My speech workbook.* (Book 4). Danville, IL: Interstate.

Powers, M. (1971). Clinical and educational procedures in functional disorders of articulation. In L. Travis (Ed.), *Handbook of speech pathology and audiology.* Englewood Cliffs, NJ: Prentice-Hall.

Subtelny, J. (1980). (Ed.) *Speech assessment and speech improvement for the hearing impaired.* Washington, DC: The Alexander Graham Bell Association for the Deaf.

West, R., & Ansberry, M. (1968). *The rehabilitation of speech.* New York: Harper & Row.

Appendix A

Procedures for Assessing Speech Sound Stimulability[1]

The procedures recommended for assessing speech sound stimulability are taken from the *CAAP: Clinical Assessment of Articulation and Phonology* (Secord and Donohue, 2002). The authors would like to thank Super Duper Publications for permission to include these procedures in Appendix A.

CAAP Stimulability Procedures

The authors suggest the following procedures for testing speech sound stimulability. The most important preliminary consideration is to get the child's complete attention. Then, before actually testing production on error sounds, teach the child to be a "good imitator." That is, identify a sound that he already says correctly in his repertoire, e.g., /p/ in "pie," and go through the following warm-up procedure. Make sure you have the child's test protocol or a stimulability form like the one provided with the *CAAP* with you because you will move directly into testing stimulability after the warm-up is finished. Proceed as follows:

Examiner says: I'm going to say a word and you say it like me. The word is "pie." Now watch how I say it, then you do it.

[1] These stimulability procedures first appeared in the *CAAP Examiner's Manual*, published in 2002 by Super Duper Publications. For more information, go to www.superduperinc.com.

Present the word in a slow and exaggerated manner so the child gets the idea of "saying it just like me (you)." This is very important because you need to train the child to imitate, especially children who often present with multiple errors. The important issue is this: Many children never quite understand that they are expected to really focus on what the examiner is doing, and then do their best to say it "just like me." This may take some training, but it is worth it. You are likely to obtain more reliable results from children who are truly "focused" on imitating, than those who, after stimulation is presented, retreat to their error response because the replacement behavior marks meaning for them. Sometimes the warm-up procedure takes a few minutes and may require challenging the child to do their best as though it was a game.

After the warm-up training is finished and the examiner is convinced the child knows how to play the imitation ("say it just like me") game, stimulability testing can begin.

The procedures for testing stimulability vary slightly based upon where and how examiners were trained. The authors recommend the following:

1. Identify the speech sounds produced in error. You may stimulate production in both the initial and final positions or choose the position known to be most favorable. For a detailed summary of favorable speech production contexts, consult Kent (1981). Normally, if a child can correctly say a sound in one position, stimulability testing is not needed.

2. Using the *CAAP* Stimulability Form (or the articulation test protocol) with the target sounds already identified, move quickly into stimulability testing because the child is "warmed up" and ready to continue the imitation game. Proceed as follows:

   Examiner says: You are so good at this. Let's do some more.

Present each word with clear articulation, holding the child's attention as before. Continue through each test word, reinforcing the child by saying such things as, "You're saying it just like me, you're watching me really well, let's do a few more," etc. The important part is to keep the child focusing on producing the sound just like you.

Should the sound not be stimulable at the word response level, the examiner can present stimulations in isolation (at the isolation-syllable level). The examiner should move to the less sophisticated response level after all the targeted sounds have been presented at the word level. Proceed as follows:

   Examiner says: Now let's say some sounds, are you watching?
                   … good!
                   Say them just like me.

Present the sound. If the sound is a nasal, fricative, or postvocalic /ɝ/ as in "her," it can be presented in isolation. If it is a stop, glide, affricate, or a liquid, it will be presented as a syllable, e.g., /pʌ/, /tʃʌ/, /lʌ/, etc. Present all targeted sounds until stimulability testing is finished.

Special Note

Be careful when there are a number of error sounds to assess because the child's attention may wane. You may need to give him a short break or switch tasks momentarily to ensure the child is completely focused on what you are doing.

Appendix B

Quick Screens of Articulation Consistency[1]

Articulation errors, especially those in young children, are often variable and inconsistent (Secord and Shine, 2003; Bernthal and Bankson, 2004). Indeed, clients often produce speech sounds correctly in some contexts, even though in others they produce those same sounds consistently in error. The value of these contextual effects is discussed in Chapter 1, for it creates a starting point for eliciting new sound behaviors.

For many years, clinicians used the *Deep Test of Articulation* (McDonald, 1964) to find phonetic contexts where children could produce their articulation errors correctly. More recently, the *S-CAT: Secord Contextual Articulation Tests* (Secord and Shine, 2003) was developed to provide a faster and more in-depth approach to contextual assessment. The quick screens of articulation consistency contained in this appendix were adapted from the *S-CAT Contextual Articulation Probes*. These probes are very short, screening-like measures that help clinicians estimate phonetic variability. Clinicians use them to find words in which the client makes sounds correctly, and ultimately, they save themselves valuable time in the treatment process. In addition, they may use the *S-CAT* materials more generally to gain an in-depth understanding of sound production processes.

The authors would like to thank Super Duper Publications for their support and permission to develop these quick screens of consistency from the *S-CAT* materials. For more information on the *S-CAT*, consult www.superduperinc.com.

A quick screen (QS) is provided for each consonant sound except /ʒ/. Each consonant QS contains 20 words in which a variety of front and back vowels systematically surround the target consonant. For consonants that initiate and terminate a word, the QS provide 10 words for both the initial and final word

---

[1] These quick screen items were adapted from the *Secord Contextual Articulation Tests (S-CAT)* published by Super Duper Publications.

positions respectively. For consonants with only one syllabic function (initiating or terminating), the QS uses all 20 words for that purpose. In addition, quick screens are provided for all monothongs and diphthongs (10 words each).

Directions for the Quick Screens

Administration of the quick screens is presented in an imitation protocol. The following format is suggested:

1. Identify the sounds in error from a standardized articulation/phonology test and observation of conversational speech.

2. Select quick screen(s) that correspond(s) to the error consonant(s) and/or vowel(s).

3. Instruct the client to imitate the target words using the following directions:

   a. Clinician: I am going to say some words. You are to say the word that I say. Listen. Say "bee."
   b. Client responds: "Bee."
   c. Clinician: "Good, you said "bee."
   d. *Note:* Repeat directions if the client has not correctly responded, and introduce trials words "bed" and "shoe."

4. Once the client is correctly following the instructions, present the target words from the appropriate (i.e., sounds that are in error) quick screen.

5. Keep records of the target words produced correctly and incorrectly.

6. Review the performance profile identifying the following patterns:

   a. Consistency of correct production
   b. Facilitating environments(the vowel and/or consonant environments in which the target sound is correctly and incorrectly produced)

7. Determine if intervention can proceed. Either utilize the facilitating environments identified in the QS, or proceed to the implementation of techniques as described in the previous chapters of this text.

Quick Screens of Articulation Consistency

/p/

peach	pool	keep	cup
pin	put	lip	soup
paid	poke	tape	hope
pet	pie	step	top
pack	pow	cap	type

/b/

beat	boot	fib	curb
big	book	rib	rub
bait	bone	web	tube
bed	ball	cab	robe
back	bite	tab	job

/t/

teeth	tune	meat	boot
tip	took	bit	put
take	toad	wait	note
ten	talk	let	caught
tack	top	hat	got

/d/

deep	dune	weed	food
dish	dome	kid	good
date	dog	made	load
deck	dot	bed	odd
dance	dine	sad	ride

/k/

keep	cool	week	duke
kiss	coat	pick	look
cane	call	lake	joke
cat	cot	deck	hawk
cup	kite	back	lock

/g/

geese	goose	league	hug
give	good	pig	bug
game	goat	leg	dog
get	gone	beg	log
gab	got	bag	fog

/s/

seen	sun	peace	goose
sit	soon	kiss	toss
safe	soap	face	dice
set	sock	guess	mouse
sat	sign	pass	choice

/z/

tease	zoo	bees	choose
zip	zoom	his	those
zane	zone	raise	jaws
zest	zombie	has	pies
zap	zero	buzz	cows

/f/

feet	foot	leaf	surf
fish	phone	if	puff
face	fall	safe	goof
fence	fox	deaf	cough
fat	fine	laugh	life

/v/

veal	van	leave	serve
visit	vote	live	love
vase	vault	gave	move
vest	voice	save	drove
verse	vine	have	dive

/θ/

thief	third	teeth	earth
thick	thirst	faith	youth
thin	thumb	death	both
theft	thought	path	moth
thank	thigh	math	mouth

/ð/

these	their	breathe	smooth
this	the	seethe	soothe
they	those	with	clothe
them	thine	bathe	loathe
that	thou	lathe	tithe

/ʃ/

sheep	shoe	leash	rush
ship	should	fish	bush
shake	show	wish	push
shell	shop	mesh	wash
shack	shine	dash	gush

/h/

heat	hat	whose	hop
his	heard	hook	high
hay	hurry	hold	how
him	hug	home	hang
head	hub	hall	huge

/tʃ/

cheek	choose	teach	lunch
chin	chose	witch	march
chase	chalk	fetch	coach
check	chop	match	watch
champ	chime	such	ouch

/dʒ/

jeep	jump	bridge	badge
jig	juice	page	large
jail	joke	cage	fudge
jet	jaw	edge	dodge
jazz	job	ledge	urge

/m/

meet	moon	team	gum
miss	mow	limb	room
made	mop	game	home
men	mice	them	Tom
match	moist	lamb	dime

/n/

need	new	seen	sun
knit	nose	win	moon
name	not	rain	phone
neck	nice	ten	gone
nut	now	can	fine

/ŋ/

king	spring	rang	kong
sing	bring	gang	strong
ring	bang	long	young
thing	sang	song	tongue
wing	hang	wrong	among

/w/

week	wag	wound	watch
win	was	wood	wire
way	won	woke	wine
wake	worm	wall	wife
wet	word	wash	wow

/j/

yeast	yell	use	yearn
yield	yank	you'll	York
yes	yam	yawn	your
year	youth	yolk	yarn
yet	you	yacht	yard

/l/

leaf	loot	feel	fool
lick	look	pill	pull
late	load	nail	hole
led	lawn	bell	call
laugh	lock	pal	mile

prevocalic	**/r/**	**postvocalic**	**/ɚ/**
read	root	bird	hair
rich	road	girl	deer
rain	wrong	bar	hear
red	rock	part	poor
ran	ride	bear	fire

vowel	**/i/**	**vowel**	**/ɪ/**
key	sheep	it	did
feet	rean	rich	fish
beet	peach	will	give
eat	week	inch	him
leaf	seat	big	lid

vowel	**/e/**	**vowel**	**/ɛ/**
gate	pain	get	men
fade	same	fresh	beg
name	lane	edge	head
race	tame	web	pet
wave	face	rent	deck

vowel	**/æ/**	**vowel**	**/u/**
math	gas	root	who
back	tag	lose	boot
rag	ran	tooth	loop
patch	dash	goose	rude
cab	sad	soon	move

vowel	**/ʊ/**	**vowel**	**/o/**
hook	should	boat	loaf
soot	good	don't	goat
put	look	road	rose
book	woof	note	vote
wool	push	close	home

vowel	**/ɔ/**	**vowel**	**/ɑ/**
paw	ball	watch	stop
chalk	talk	top	wand
lawn	cough	shock	job
sought	off	doll	lot
fall	long	shop	dock

vowel	**/ʌ/**	**vowel**	**/ə/**
just	rough	sofa	ago
love	muck	soda	alike
cut	once	across	above
rub	come	complete	china
from	done	famous	open

diphthong	**/au/**	**diphthong**	**/ai/**
out	hour	might	mike
mouse	cow	kite	guide
now	sow	time	fine
loud	noun	five	light
brown	town	white	time

diphthong	**/ɔɪ/**
boy	joy
voice	toys
coil	noise
coin	poise
join	boil

Appendix C

An Elicitation Strategy for Clients Who Lisp

Richard E. Shine
East Carolina University

Introduction

Eliciting correct sound behaviors in children who lisp is often a real challenge for speech-language pathologists (SLPs). The challenge comes from the fact that an auditory approach (e.g., use of an exact auditory model of the /s/ sound in early treatment) is often unsuccessful. Despite the clinician's best attempts to break down the auditory commands into a step-by-step elicitation process, the error responses persist. They continue even though the child can hear (discriminate) the difference between the error sound and a correct /s/ production. Two reasons for this appear to be (1) the habit strength of the error sound behaviors (i.e., although the /s/ sound is acquired as early as age 3, many children who lisp do not receive treatment until well into their school-age years), and (2) the error sound itself (e.g., the /s/ approximation in children who lisp marks or codes meaning for the child). So in the child's understanding, one doesn't "see" with eyes, but one does "~s~ee" with eyes (~x~ = distortion of /s/ as a lateral, frontal, or interdental lisp). The child with a lisp can hear the difference between the /s/ and the lateral, frontal, or interdental "~s~", but the meaning is carried by "~s~". Hence, the clinician's use of an auditory model will have limited impact, and it may actually interfere with the elicitation process.

In addressing this problem, you may experience greater success by using a sound the child produces correctly that shares features with the error sound, or by "tricking" the child into believing that his new target sound is something other than the error sound. With clients who lisp, and in particular, the child with a lateral lisp, this strategy can produce positive results almost immediately.

To be effective, the clinician must literally stop talking about the /s/ and /z/ sounds and focus the child's attention on a new target. Start by having the child produce a new sound, an isolated, prolonged "t" sound. Show the child how to produce this new sound (1) with a duration of at least three to four seconds, (2) with obvious aspiration, and, (3) with a **bite-block**[1] in place between the child's teeth. The frication of the prolonged "t" is characteristic of a "tssssssss"; but because of the open bite created by the bite-block placement, the "s" is acoustically and physiologically different and is not recognized by the child as an /s/. If during your modeling or the child's production, he or she concludes that the prolonged, fricated sound is an /s/, the client will immediately access his phonologic knowledge base and produce his error phone (i.e., a lateral, frontal, or interdental lisp). Thus, it is important to give the "new target sound" a fictitious label, such as a "German tee." Then, provide consistent ongoing verbal feedback in response to the child's productions of this new sound, and avoid any and all use of the /s/ and /z/ sounds as models.

A step-by-step sample sequence of this elicitation procedure is presented in detail below.

Types of Lisps

The following discussion covers the types of lisps: frontal lisp, interdental lisp, and lateral lisp.

Type 1: The Frontal Lisp

Feature characteristics (see Figure C.1):

- Teeth are not together (approximated), blade of tongue is near the cutting edge of the upper central incisors with the tip typically near or behind the lower central incisors. Tongue is not between the teeth as with an interdental lisp.

- Distorted release of air over the tongue toward the cutting edges of upper central incisors. The stridency feature is distorted and the degree of stridency is possibly reduced

- Velum closed

- Vocal folds silent

[1] See Figures C.3 and C.4.

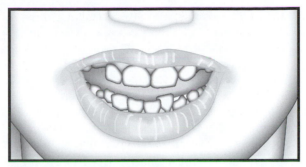

Figure C.1 Frontal lisp

The fontal lisp typically involves only the /s/ and /z/ sounds; however, some children also distort phonetically similar sounds, such as /ʃ, ʒ, tʃ, dʒ/, which they produce without the teeth together (approximated) and/or with incorrect tongue placement. Sometimes children with an open bite exhibit a frontal lisp; but other individuals with an open bite appear to lisp because of the visibility of the tongue. However, by carefully observing tongue placement with a penlight, you can evaluate the correctness of the placement and the production of /s/ and /z/. Another client group erroneously identified as having a frontal lisp is young children who are missing their upper central incisors. The visibility of the tongue and the modified acoustic production resulting from the missing teeth can result in the misdiagnosis. When the teeth eventually erupt, the misdiagnosis will become more obvious.

Type 2: The Interdental Lisp

Feature characteristics:

- The tip of the tongue is protruded between the upper and lower incisors/teeth, lightly contacting them.

- The body of the tongue is relatively flat.

- Distorted air is forced through the space between the tongue and upper front teeth.

- The stridency feature is distorted.

Like the frontal lisp, the interdental lisp typically involves only the /s/ and /z/ sounds; however, some children exhibit a distortion of phonetically similar sounds, such as /ʃ, ʒ, tʃ, dʒ/. These errors usually occur when they are produced without the teeth together (approximated) and/or when there is incorrect tongue placement. See Figure C.2.

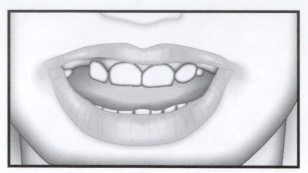

Figure C.2 Interdental lisp

The sound is typically but erroneously referred to as a /θ/ for /s/ and /ð/ for /z/ substitution because of the interdental placement. However, acoustic analysis of the error phone reveals the presence of stridency; thus, the substitution is a phonetic distortion of either the /s/ or /z/ sound. The correct production of the voiceless /θ/ and the voiced /ð/ sounds do not include the stridency feature.

Type 3: The Lateral Lisp

Feature characteristics:

- Tongue tip touching the alveolar ridge
- Voiceless air stream passing over the sides of the tongue
- Air forced laterally creating significantly distorted frication
- Velum closed
- Vocal folds silent

Like other types of lisps, the lateral lisp typically affects the /s/ and /z/ sounds, but there is almost always a distortion of phonetically similar sounds, including /ʃ, ʒ, tʃ, dʒ/. The lateral /s/ error pattern is usually consistent in all contexts that include these sounds. Typically, the lateral lisp is one of the most difficult articulation errors to correct. Clinicians often agonize over the hours they have spent trying to elicit correct production. However, if a child is able to produce an aspirated /t/ sound, there is significant reason to be optimistic: the child should be able to say /s/ correctly immediately or within 10 to 20 minutes of instruction. If the child is unable to produce an aspirated /t/, then the first step in the process will be to teach him to do so (see step 1 on the following page). The elicitation strategies described here can be used with all three types of lisps, as well as with a majority of other error sounds. However, given the troublesome nature of /s/ sounds, the explanation will focus on the lateral /s/ lisp.

Step-by-Step Elicitation Procedure for the Lateral /s/ Lisp

1. Show the Child How to Use a Bite-Block

    Initiate the elicitation procedure by teaching the child to use a bite-block while producing the target sound. A bite-block is the child's sanitized thumb (see Figure C.3) or a sterile object, such as three tongue depressors stacked together (see Figure C.4). The child places the bite-block in the corner of the mouth between the molars. Use your gloved thumb or some stacked tongue depressors as your bite-block when modeling sounds for the child. The bite-block stabilizes the jaw and separates the central incisors approximately a quarter-inch (similar to an "open bite"). Stabilizing the jaw enables the child to use tongue movement patterns independent of jaw movements and typically facilitates enhanced awareness of movement and placement patterns during elicitation procedures. In addition, with the stabilized open bite, you can use a penlight to observe the movements and placement of the tongue during target sound production for lisps and other error sounds. The child's thumb is a convenient tool as it is "almost always" available for the child to place between the teeth.

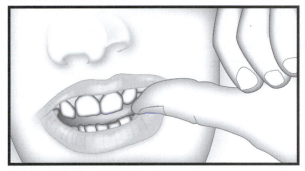

Figure C.3 Thumb bite block

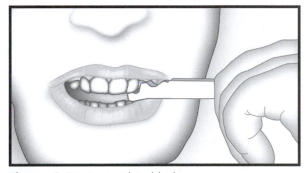

Figure C.4 Instrument bite block

2.   **Show the Child How to Produce an Aspirated "t" with a Bite-Block**

Have the child produce an isolated /t/ sound. If the "t" is aspirated, frication will be present during the explosion, suggesting that the child can produce the acoustic parameters of /s/. As a result, he or she will rarely have difficulties correcting the lateral lisp. If the child produces an unaspirated "t" (one that lacks frication), you will need to elicit and stabilize an aspirated "t" with a bite-block before moving to the next step. The unaspirated "t" may be characterized by a tongue placement that is marginally posterior to the alveolar ridge or that appears to be produced with a vowel ("tu" as in "cut"). Model the production of /t/ with your bite-block in place and with obvious aspiration. Teach an aspirated "t" without letting the child know that the eventual target sound will be a prolonged /s/ as in "tsssss." Have the child repeat the aspirated "t" several times with the bite-block to stabilize production.

3.   **Teach the New Sound: The "German, French or Long Tee" with a Bite-Block**

Instruct the child that you are going to teach him or her to say a new sound. Tell the child that the new sound is a "German tee" (or a label appropriate for your child). Model the target with your bite-block in place, and instruct the child to repeat the model with a bite-block in place. Produce five to six staccato, aspirated "t t t t t t" sounds, and prolong the last sound: "t t t t t tsssss." Once the child can imitate the model and produce a correct "tsssssss" with the bite-block in place, initiate procedures to stabilize the correct production. Have the child say "t t t t t tsssss," take a breath, and immediately say it again. Repeat this five or six times, and then take a 10- to 15-second rest break. Repeat the same procedure several times until you feel confident that the production is stable.

Note that you must provide significant verbal feedback about the correctness/incorrectness of the child's responses. Emphasize placement and tactile awareness. For correct responses, you might say the following:

- "Great, your tongue is touching behind your front teeth"
- "Great, feel where your tongue is"
- "Awesome, where's your tongue?"
- "Super, your tongue is up high, right here behind your teeth." (Touch the child's upper lip beneath the nose.)
- "Awesome 'tssssss' sound." (Provide a model with your bite-block in place.)

For incorrect responses you might say:

- "No, you didn't bite down."
- "No, that's not a German tee."

Keep in mind that the sound being produced is the "German tee" ("tssssss"), and not /s/ or /ts/. At this point in the process of establishing and stabilizing the "tssssss," I've had children remark, "Oh, I know what you're trying to do. You're trying to get me to say /s/." In so doing, the child usually reverts to the lateral "~s~" production. You should continue to assure the child that the target is the "German tee" (a new sound) and not the /s/ as we know it. For clients who read, you may have to create a fabricated grapheme to represent the "German tee" sound; and later, during the stabilization and generalization, provide printed nonsense words ending with the "German tee" ("kee tx").

4. ## Teach the Child to Produce "t t t t t tssssss" and "tssssss" with Teeth Together

    Provide a model of the "German tee" ("t t t t t tssssss") with your bite-block in place, and instruct the child to put his or her teeth together and say "t t t t t tssssss." If the child thinks he or she is producing a "German tee," he or she will almost always produce an acoustically perfect "t t t t t tssssss" with teeth together. You will hear a correct /s/ as part of the long /ts/ production. Tell the child, "That's a perfect "German tee." Then, instruct the child to say it again. Continue to model the "t t t t t tssss" with either your bite block in place or with your teeth separated at least a quarter of an inch when your bite-block is not in place.

    Next, introduce the "tsssss" production without the /t/ repetitions. Model "tsssss" with your bite block, and have the child repeat "tsssss" several times with his or her bite-block in place. Stabilize production before moving to the next step. At this point, do not be in a rush to generalize production of the new sound. Take some extra time to ensure that production is stable. Provide verbal feedback and supportive procedures for stabilization, as in step 3. *Remember:* Never provide an auditory model with your teeth together, and never let the child know that the target is /s/, because the child will typically revert to the lateral /s/ production.

    For children who do not produce the "tttttssss" sound correctly without the bite-block, it generally takes only a limited amount of instruction to elicit correct production with the teeth together. Determine what changes the child made to produce the sound incorrectly, and make changes to correct the production based on the bite-block production. Occasionally, children revert to a lateral lisp when they put their teeth back together. So if you say, "That's not a 'German tee,'" the child will almost always self-correct and repeat the "German tee" correctly. If the lateral lisp continues, return to the use of a bite-block in step 3, and complete additional stabilization procedures before continuing to step 4.

5. ## Teach Production of the "keet t t t tssssss" Nonsense Context with a Bite-Block

    For this step, if the child misarticulates /k/, you'll need to use a different consonant. Avoid using a consonant that results in a recognizable word because that will typically stimulate production of the lateral lisp.

    Start by providing a model of "keet t t t tssssss" with your bite-block in place. Ask the child to repeat the context with a bite-block in place. Continue to model the correct production and have the child repeat the context several times to stabilize production. Provide pertinent verbal feed-back for each production. Once the child stabilizes production, model the context with your bite-block in place, but instruct the child to put the teeth together without the bite-block and say the context: "keet t t t t tsssss." Repeat the practice several times to stabilize production.

Once the child stabilizes production, model the context "keetsssss" (eliminate the "t" repetitions) with your bite-block in place, but instruct the child to repeat the context with teeth together, without the bite-block. Finally, model the context "keetsssss" with your bite-block in place for only the "tssss" part, and instruct the child to produce the context "keetsssss" with teeth together for only the "tssss." Model the response by holding your bite-block (thumb or stacked tongue depressors) near the corner of your mouth, initiating production of the context "kee," quickly slipping the bite-block between the molars, and biting down to produce the "tssss." Always use the bite-block or open bite to provide the model. Take your time to automate the child's production before moving to next step.

6.   Generalize Production of the "tssss" to Other Contexts

Introduce a wide variety of other nonsense contexts. Begin with high front vowels, and use only consonants that the child can produce correctly. Generally, once the "base" context "keetsssss" is stabilized with the child's teeth together for only the "tssssss," you can add many new contexts quickly. The following words should be appropriate for most children: geets, heets, deets, weets, bits, nits, fets, hets, and bots. If the child produces a lateral lisp in the production of any context, provide verbal feedback ("No that's not your "German tee!"), eliminate that context, and move to the next word in your list. Do not attempt to correct the production.

7.   Teach "I have a 'keetsss'" with the Teeth Together Only on the "tsss"

Model the sentence "I have a 'keetssss'" with your bite-block in place or your teeth apart. Ask the child to repeat the sentence several times with teeth together on the "German tee" only. Some children need to practice putting their teeth together for the whole word "keetsss" before putting their teeth together for only the "tssss." Provide significant verbal feedback about the correctness/incorrectness of each response. Remember to coach the child. Stabilize the production before moving on to next step.

8.   Generalize Production of Other Nonsense Contexts with Teeth Together only on "tsss"

Introduce new sentences using a variety of contexts:

- "The keetsss can fly."
- "I like deetsss."
- "Feetsss can be funny."
- "I ate weetssss for lunch."

Model the sentence with your bite-block in place, using a wide variety of sentences and contexts. The child puts teeth together only on the "tsss."

At this point, you may want to assess the child's use of the rule for plurality in the production of "keetsss." Ask the child to say, "I have *three* keetssss." With the mention of this phonological rule (plural marker), you can expect the lateral lisp to occur. Follow-up by having the child say, "I have *one* "keetsssss," and the "tsss" will again be correctly produced. This usually suggests that the child is still using the lateral lisp /s/ rule to code plurality and the "German tee" to code the notion of singular. The results suggest that the child is very capable of producing a correct /s/ in /ts/; but the child continues to use the rules for the lateral lisp with real words during most speaking situations. Generalizing the correct sound to all /s/ contexts, including real words, can begin by making the child aware of his or her different productions for "one keets" and "three keet~s~." Make the child aware that the production of the "German tee" includes the correct /s/ sound. Show the child a picture of cats and ask, "What are these?" The child will typically say "cats" with a lateral lisp. If the child is instructed to produce "cats" with a "German tee" he or she will generally produce a correct /ts/ or will quickly respond to the bite-block and teeth-together instructions to produce a correct /ts/ in "cats." At this point, most children are able to produce both their old sound (lateral "~s~") and the new sound (German tee" /ts/) in most word-final /ts/ words, following your instruction. Now they are ready to work on word-initial /s/ contexts. One should also expect the child to spontaneously generalize the correct /s/ production in spontaneous speech.

9. Generalize Production of the Word-Final /ts/ Cluster to the Word-Initial /s/

Develop bisyllable contexts to transfer the correct production of "ts" in "keets" to the /s/ in words beginning with vowels. In effect, add the prepositions *in, on, up, under, over, out* to the end of the "keets" sound. The words "under" and "over" may be inappropriate for children with post-vocalic /ɚ/ misarticulations but only if the contexts result in misarticulation of /s/. Pair the word "keets" (teeth together on the "ts") with the prepositions, and have the child produce two-word utterances, such as "keets in," in a conversational manner. This will facilitate correct production of a word-initial /s/ (e.g., "keetss-sin"). The inclusion of the /s/ in "sin" will occur automatically; and with repeated productions, the child generally develops appropriate patterns to produce word-initial /s/ sounds correctly in other contexts.

To create visual representations of these nonsense phrases, draw a nonsense picture of a "keets" (an animal, a monster, or a unique design) on a small card. You will also need a cup, a block, and a small chair, or similar objects. Have the child hold the picture of "keets" in one hand and place the picture in a cup. As the child does so, model "keetss-sin" by stating: "You put 'keetss-sin' the cup!" The /s/ in "ts" is "just barely" prolonged, and there is no pause between the words. Strong linguistic stress is placed on the word "in." You may want to experiment with linguistic stress. Stress on the second syllable facilitates correction production of /s/ for most children, but some do better with stress on the first syllable or near-equal stress on both syllables. In addition, carefully monitor your model to ensure that the /s/ in "sin" is produced naturally, rather than being stressed or exaggerated. Have the child place the picture in the cup two or three times while you say "keetss-sin." Finally instruct the child to say "keetss-sin" as he or she places the picture in the cup. The child will be saying the context correctly with no apparent awareness of the correct /s/ in "sin." Have the child verbalize in the same manner while placing or putting "keets on" (the block), "up" (in the air), "under" (the chair), "over" (the cup), and "out" (the door). Stabilize production in each of the contexts, and gradually add real and nonsense words to develop new contexts, using only sounds the child produces correctly: (1) beets, feets, pits, mates, pats, boats, boots; (2) eat, it, ape, Abe, egg, oat, oom.

As an alternate strategy, combine words that end in /t/ with words that begin with /s/, such as "beet soup." Have the child practice saying "beet" with an aspirated "t." With your bite-block in place, model "beet soup," and instruct the child to repeat the context with teeth together on the /t/ sound. The pattern frequently facilitates correct production of the /s/ in "soup" with children who have completed steps 8 and 9 above, and it can be used with many new words to enhance generalization. This is not surprising, given that when "beat soup" is produced correctly in conversational speech, "soup" becomes "tsoup." In addition, phonetic analysis reveals that when produced conversationally in the bisyllable context "keets-in," the /s/ in the word "sin" is actually a /ts/ (e.g., "keet-tsin"). This phonetic change appears to be an area for future research related to articulation therapy.

Once the child has completed the nine steps above, introduce additional generalization procedures as necessary. Typically, generalization to conversational speech should occur rapidly, because coarticulatory patterns were used to elicit correct production, and because the child recognizes and self-corrects most of the /s/ misarticulations. If the child lateralizes production of other fricative and affricative sounds, the step-by-step process using the bite-block and penlight is generally an effective approach.

Conclusion

As Dr. Van Riper stated in his letter to Dr. Secord at the beginning of this book: "I constantly urged my students to develop better methods of their own." In similar words, my mentor at Penn State, Dr. Eugene McDonald, expressed the same message many times. *Eliciting Sounds, Second Edition,* blends science and practice in a way that was not available to earlier generations of speech clinicians. I grew up learning the science as best I could, but I learned that practice is often an elegant mix of science, motivation, and heart. I encourage you to incorporate all three.